The Fabulous Girl's Guide to Being Fearless

What every girl should know

By

Cathy Steinberg

Dedication

This book is dedicated to my Eden.

May your life be full of love, happiness, and peace.

I love you with all my heart –

Mommy

Mami, Siempre en my Corazon.

Special dedication to the memory of all
the girls who didn't make it home...

Published by White Feather Press, LLC
www.whitefeatherpress.com

ISBN: 978-1-61808-053-0
Printed in the United States of America

Cover design created by Cathy Steinberg

White Feather Press

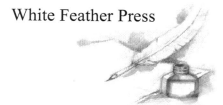

Reaffirming Faith in God, Family, and Country!

Contents

Overview

FBI statistics show 1 in 4 women will be the victim of a crime in their lifetime. A staggering number of those crimes will result in extreme violence and death. Victimization is a life-altering experience that changes a woman's world forever. A woman needs to be aware of the danger she faces, be prepared to escape, and be willing to defend her life with strength and conviction in order to survive....thereby becoming FEARLESS while keeping her Fabulous life intact.

Introduction

"*Ruuun Cathy*" is all I could muster the courage to tell myself. Get away. Go. My little body frozen in fear could do nothing but tremble. There was no escaping him. I didn't know what to do and was I helpless. There was a monster in my life. He was shameless, evil, and would stop at nothing to hurt me and others. I will forever live with the nightmare of the loss of my innocent and peaceful existence.

> *"Crime butchers innocence to secure a throne, and innocence struggles with all its might against the attempts of crime."*
>
> *– Maximilien Robespierre*

The moment I discovered self-defense I knew I would NEVER be a helpless victim ever again. I also knew I would be dedicating my life to helping YOU keep your innocent and blissful existence intact. I think you are Fabulous. You are entitled to live in safety and security while enjoying a wonderful life, and I'm going to help guide you through the journey toward that goal.

> *"We gain strength, and courage, and confidence by each experience in which we really stop to look fear in the face... we must do that which we think we cannot"*
>
> *- Eleanor Roosevelt*

I spent years working in prisons to meet in person the creepy monsters, the crazies, and degenerates who want to hurt you. I became obsessed with learning their patterns of behavior, their motives, and how they choose their victims. What I initially learned about their twisted minds caused me to spiral into darkness and fear. I struggled to find a path to understanding. Going in, I never imagined that what I would learn about these men and women would be so disturbing. I frequently say that I used to think movies exaggerated crime stories. I now realize the real-life monster dwarfs anything I ever saw in movies. I often wondered, what if their victims were prepared to deal with these kinds of monsters? What if they knew how to help themselves? To not just survive, but to win. How can I make a difference?

One particular beast I often spoke to enjoyed terrorizing his victims. He derived so much pleasure in the fear he inflicted upon his prey. It was him who made me decide to stay longer and work harder at gaining the knowledge I needed to help you be safe. His sentence will someday come to an end and he will one day be a free man. I realized he will never stop. His mind was wired wrong and prison was no deterrent for him. I can help you understand there are people who don't think like you or me. Theirs is an ugly and sick reality that needs to be addressed in order for you to stay one step ahead of them. You matter. Your safety matters. Most of all, your peace of mind matters. This book is about empowerment, not fear.

There are a few things you need to learn, understand, and practice to make your transition to

Fearless happen. Situational awareness is a term used to describe the ability to understand what is going on around you, quickly process the information, and act accordingly to produce a positive outcome. In your case: Get away safely.

The following alert levels are important in training your awareness to identify a bad situation before it becomes a threat. Developed by Jeff Cooper, as what he calls the "combat mindset," it is still the best way to describe the different levels of mental alert for any situation.

- ♩ ***White Alert*** – You've got other things on your mind. You are distracted, unaware, and unsuspecting of any surprises that may come your way. You are searching for your keys or texting instead of paying attention to your surroundings. You're not thinking about your environment while you walk around. If attacked, you will certainly be caught off guard at this level of awareness. At White Alert your only chance to get away will be if your beast is a complete idiot or drunk. Remember, attackers are looking for women in their white alert mode. You are an easy target and that is what they are looking for. Actually, it's what they are hoping for.

- ♩ ***Pink Alert*** – You are alert and aware. You are ready for all possibilities. You use all your senses of awareness. Your eyes and ears are scanning your surroundings and your intuition is turned on. You are up to date with current events and know that possible danger is lurking about. You carry yourself in a manner that lets everyone know you are alert and aware of everything happening around you. You are in F.A.B. (Focused, Aware, Brave) mode, have confidence — and it shows. Technically, it is yellow alert but pink is fabulous. This is the mental state you should be in at all times until it is time to escalate.

✓ **Orange Alert** – You've picked up on something suspicious. A staring man prowling around has made you nervous. You instantly start thinking of ways to get away but know that defending yourself is a possibility. You are confident and focused. You see every method of escape or every weapon at your disposal clearly. You are in reaction mode and ready. You keep your alert level up until the threat is gone or you have left the area and are safe.

✓ **Red Alert** – This is where the threat is upon you. Your safe zone has been crossed and you have to immediately act. It is here and now that you cannot waste a second. You are screaming to get attention, running away, and quickly reaching for a weapon. You are in the moment of the event and have to escape. Your only objective is to save yourself and get away no matter what it takes.

An important thought to keep in mind is this: A predator is looking for easy prey. An unaware victim can be easily overwhelmed by surprise attack. Not you; awareness and vigilance will become second nature. By the end of this book you will be transformed from fabulous to Fearlessly Fabulous.

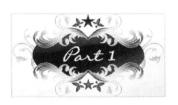

You are Fabulous!

The dictionary defines the word Fabulous as amazingly or almost unbelievably great or impressive, described in or typical of myths and legends, extremely good, pleasant, or enjoyable — all of which describes you perfectly. I think you are Fabulous! Women have an inner strength and beauty that cannot be described. Words fail to explain the depth of a woman's heart and soul.

We are all Fabulous in our own special way. Every part of you radiates your own unique brand of fabulous.

This book is my gift to you, Fabulous, because my hope is that you continue to live free from fear and get a chance to fully live up to the wonder that you are — the extraordinary, amazingly magnificent you.

"Love is a fruit in season at all times, and within reach of every hand"

-Mother Teresa

Fabulous Girl Dating

As a Fabulous girl you socialize regularly, have great self-esteem, and your dating options are wide open. You are breezy and fun. Being awesome is just in your nature. Some guy would be lucky to have such a fabulous girl like you in his life.

You are never one to settle for second best, so when you decide you would like to start dating, you take your time to find an amazing, kind, and wonderful guy for you. Dating and finding your Mr. Right is an exciting adventure. You are going to enjoy the ride and not worry about anything. The right guy is out there waiting just for you. He will be your perfect match, so remember not to waste your precious energy on Mr. Wrong. Mr. Right will come along when it is time. Enjoy your life and wonderful friends. Meet new people and stay Fabulous!

When you are out meeting new guys and dating, here are some tips:

- When meeting someone new, give them a Favicard instead of your number. Favicards are your social networking cards.
- Always tell a friend where you are going.
- Offer to meet a first date at the date location.
- Snap a picture of your date and send it to a friend.
- Never let a date put you down.
- Be treated like a lady, nothing less will do.
- Know when to say "NEXT!".

Favi-fabulous

You enjoy meeting new people and are now actively dating. On a fun night out you happen to meet a handsome stranger. He asks you for your number, and being the savvy girl you are, you whip out your chic Favicard instead of trying to scream your number or (preferably) your email address over the loud music. Favicards are your social networking cards. You could customize your cards with a cool graphic on one side and your contact info on the other. The absolute best benefit is that you could stylishly give him your email contact information and if he turns out to be creepy, just block his emails without batting an eye. You've saved yourself the trouble of having to change your number because Mr. Creepy is calling you at all hours. Ewww. A girl needs her beauty sleep, not to be annoyed in the middle of the night by a stalker.

Your bestie knows best

Every one of us has that one special girlfriend. She

has been with you through good times and bad. She knows when you had your first kiss, your first crush, as well as your first date. She is always there for you. She is your bestie. Your bestie knows everything about you. She knows you like a sister and when it comes to dating someone new, tell her everything. If you are going to be spending time getting to know a stranger, telling your bestie all about him will help keep you safe.

When planning a night out with a new mystery man, always tell her (and another friend or relative) where you are going. You are a smart girl, always thinking ahead about all the possibilities. Your bestie will be a good resource to help locate you if something happens, or if you are left stranded and in need of a way home.

Secrets will work against you in an emergency; so gossip away, Fabulous! This is one of those times when gossiping is good!

Have car will drive

A rule you should follow for the few first dates with your new mystery guy is: drive yourself. While it may seem romantic to have a charming guy come to your house and sweep you off your feet for a lovely evening, this isn't the movies. In real life, that cute charismatic guy could be a wolf in sheep's clothing.   Don't have a stranger come to your home. Take your time. Get to know him first. The exciting part about meeting someone new is discovering all the cool things about this mysterious new person. Sometimes it turns out good and sometimes bad. Keeping your home and other personal information about yourself private is an absolute must until your new guy has proven himself worthy.

My girlfriend, Lily, once met a guy at a club on one of our girl's nights out. I must admit he was handsome and fascinating. They sat and chatted at the bar for some time. After a few drinks, she gave him her number and we left. He called her the next day (double points for not playing the wait-3-days-to-call game). They set up a date a few nights later. He came to her house and picked her up. During the date he started to act weird. She said he made some dirty remarks and made her feel uncomfortable. Lily cut the date short and asked him to take her home. While in the car, he made a few more inappropriate comments that made her really nervous.

Lily immediately found herself looking for a way out. She ended up getting out of the car at a stop light by a coffee shop she knew well and called a friend to pick her up. Mr. Creepy spent the next several days calling and texting her repeatedly. She also noticed his car parked down the street from her home the following week. Needless to say, she was terrified for quite some time afterwards.

Do not trust a pretty face until you get to know the real person. Drive yourself to your first dates. Don't invite a potential monster into your home. Keep your home your safe zone. Make it a strictly VIP only spot.

The Sly Paparazzi

Another good habit while out on a first date is to snap a picture of your guy and send it to a friend. You are a crafty girl and a smooth talker, so snapping his picture should be a breeze. It's a smart move to do for safety while he thinks you're just quirky. I claim to be paparazzi-esque early on in my conversations, before any date with my potential new guy, so when I do pull out the phone for a quick snap shot, he thinks I'm just being me. I'm five steps ahead of him and he doesn't even know it. That picture could be valuable if you don't make it home. The police will have the face and name of the last person who was with you. Along with where you were last and what your companion was wearing. If they go to interview the staff at the location, that picture of him, looking exactly the same and wearing the same thing he wore, will help jar memories better than any verbal description or old picture could do. It could save your life. So snap away, sly paparazzi! Thinking quick and on your feet is a habit you will learn with practice. Being wise and planning ahead could possibly save your life.

Know when to say "Next!"

Isn't it frequently the case, as women, that we try to a) make things better, b) fix things in our relationship, or c) change Mr. Wrong to Mr. Right? The rational voice inside our head is screaming for us to leave him, but the beating of our romantic heart is too loud for us to hear it. Learning how to lower the volume on your love-sick heart will let your voice of reason steer you away from wasting your time in a potentially bad or dangerous relationship. You deserve better, but you need to realize it. No one can do that for you.

"Don't you dare, for one more second, surround yourself with people who are not aware of the greatness that you are"

Jo Blackwell-Preston

If a guy you are dating makes a hurtful comment to

you or about you, shut him down quickly. You should ALWAYS be treated respectfully and like a lady. Anything less will not do. There aren't enough excuses in the world to allow a man to mistreat you. You are secure enough to get away from the situation if the need arises. Remember that you are awesome. If you are dating someone who doesn't appreciate your awesomeness, move on.

As a Fabulous girl you should trust your intuition. You are training yourself to have a sharp instinct and cat-like response. If you have a feeling, (you know the one – it's the little voice in your head or the sinking feeling in your stomach) pay attention to it. Mr. Wrong always leaves clues. There really is no mystery. A common mistake is to ignore the warning signs. Too often we make excuses for poor behavior instead of seeing it for what it really is: a sure sign that he is not the one. We walk around with blinders on, and those blinders cloud our judgment in other situations as well. If you grow accustomed to ignoring the bad behavior of those closest to you, you will miss the clues when you encounter a potential threat.

Your internal "jerk identification system" needs to be used frequently in order to be finely tuned. Tear off those blinders and replace them with sharp awareness. You will see every circumstance for what it is, whether it is with a boyfriend or a stranger on the street. Once properly identified, you can effectively deal with the situation, no matter how bad it is.

"Love yourself and treat yourself with dignity, and others will do the same."

The right man in your life is kind. He does not put himself before you. He doesn't make you nervous (in a bad way, not the sweet-butterflies-in-your-stomach nervous) when he is around. His conduct doesn't constantly have you making excuses to others for his poor behavior. He doesn't continually stress you out and make you sick to your stomach. He is hospitable and courteous to your family. When you are out together with friends he is sociable, mingles, and takes part in the gathering. Don't settle. Good and considerate men are out there waiting for a Fabulous girl like you.

One Saturday while lazily floating in the pool, I over-heard a spirited conversation a girl was having poolside on her phone. I'm not an eavesdropper, but she was very loudly and rudely killing my mojo with her noisy complaining. After a few minutes of listening, my anger turned to sympathy. She was talking about her boyfriend to a friend, telling her how they were fighting and how he hates her friends and some family members. She ex-pressed grief about having given up so much for him by cutting off contact with a few friends he disapproved of and not speaking to her male friends anymore, yet he was still not happy. She griped about his unrelenting con-trolling and critical behavior. He raised his voice and yelled at her often, she lamented. Listening to her reveal story after story about the poor way he treated her and how she didn't know what to do to make him happy, made me what to jump up and knock some sense into her. It isn't supposed to be that hard. The right guy for you isn't going to demand anything so ridiculous

I have come to believe that caring for myself is not self indulgency, Car-ing for myself is an act of self-preservation.

Audre Lorde

of you. He trusts and values you as an equal and wouldn't demand you stop speaking to friends and family. Trust me when I say I have been guilty of putting up with Mr. Wrong, too. But identifying the situation in your relationship, and knowing when it is not right for you, is vital to building self esteem and confidence. Only by standing up for yourself will you really start to reclaim your magnificence. Have you ever allowed a man to mistreat while you sat back and let it happen by justifying his behavior?

Realize this: if you tolerate yourself being treated poorly, it becomes your norm. You are in an emotional white alert mode. When a stranger begins displaying the subtle warning before he attacks, you will not realize it until it's too late. Take a stand and rid yourself of any guy who doesn't respect you 100%. Get back to you and your happiness.

The Cheater

Hi, my name is Cathy and I have been a victim of "The Cheater". Admitting that is hard for me. I like to think of myself as a strong, confident woman. It happens to the best of us. It is our response to the cheater that determines how strong we really are. My hope is that you could avoid this person entirely, but if you happen to fall prey, then quickly recognizing it, and correcting the situation is what truly makes you strong.

My story goes like this... I met Evan at work. He was aggressive and arrogant (everything in a man you should probably avoid) and drew me in like a moth to a flame. He wasn't conceited all the time; he did have a vulnerable soft side. Actually, to describe it as a soft side is kind of misleading; it was more of a manipulative streak. He had a way with words and emotions. Playing games with women was a pastime for him. Shamefully, I too was sucked into his game. His phone rang 24/7, at all hours. He ignored some and other times grabbed his phone and would hastily go somewhere private to chat. Like a fool, I soon found myself looking at his phone, writing down numbers, and calling women who were calling him. It turns out he was dating three other women aside from me. When I confronted him he just laughed at me. I was upset with myself for ignoring the clues, like the constant phone calls when we were together and how he was never spontaneous because his time was limited.

The Cheater's main objective is to boost his ego while tearing down your confidence. Your reaction to this man is what will set you on the path to self love or low self esteem. You are Fabulous and would never tolerate being someone's second (or third) best. You should be someone's Number 1, or nothing. It will be *his* loss!

"Let men tremble to win the hand of a woman, unless they win along with it the utmost passion of her heart"
- Nathaniel Hawthorne

Hit me with your best shot!

You deserve to be cherished and respected. You will never accept anyone lifting a hand to you. Love does not work that way. Under no circumstance is violence against you ever OK. There aren't enough excuses in the world to justify any form of violence in your relationship. Let me let you in on a little secret. If you allow it to happen once, it will happen again — maybe not in the same form, perhaps different or worse, but in one way or another it will happen again. The first strike is designed to test you, to see how you will react and what you will do. The goal is to ultimately break down your confidence. Not you! Not anymore. Regaining your strength is all in your response. If you leave him, you win. If you stay, little by little your self esteem will be deflated. Your Fabulous glow will dim. Once you accept being treated like this by him, you risk being the victim of others as well. Be unwavering in your self love. You are wonderful and strong and fearless. You deserve better. Actually, you deserve the best.

Knowing when to say "Next!"

Here is the breakdown:

If he does any one of the following:

- Stands you up
- Acts creepy or makes you uncomfortable
- Makes mean or rude comments
- Doesn't communicate with you properly
- Doesn't make you happy
- Doesn't make you laugh
- Doubts how wonderful you are
- Makes you feel like you are to blame for problems
- Cheats
- EVER raises a hand to you – shoving, pushing or throwing something at you

say *"Next!"*

Relationships should be easy breezy. When the two halves fit, everything else is in harmony. There are so many wonderful guys out there waiting to meet you and have a wonderful girl like you in their life. You're building your confidence to FEARLESS level. And being Fearless means you're not afraid to expect the best for yourself, to feel confident, to feel secure, and to make necessary changes to get it.

Life is an open book in social media. It is as open as you allow for it to be – but be careful Fabulous girl! The internet never forgets!

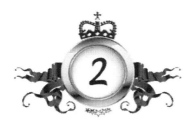

The Busy Girl's Dating System

Online Dating and Social Media Networking

For a busy girl like you, who's always on the go, online dating and socializing are a great alternative to the night club dating scene. You're ambitiously juggling work and a social calendar all in one place. Online you are in complete control of who you want to get to know and who you want to delete. You are in total control. When you have made your choice (or choices), having a plan on how to meet is crucial to being safe.

Here are some Fabulous tips:

- Don't trust the pictures.
- Have a lengthy email exchange before meeting.
- Don't send him sexy pictures.
- Don't give out your number.
- Make your first date a quickie "Meet and Greet".
- Keep your address and other personal information strictly VIP.
- Always tell a friend where you are going and call them when you leave.

In the world of online dating there is one guarantee...never trust the pictures. When it comes to pictures, everyone wants to always put their best face forward. Sometimes the picture of that face was from 10 years ago. I once met a guy online who had a couple semi-blurry pictures on his profile and a really great professional modeling shot. He looked like David Copperfield. Don't judge me! I have a weakness for mysterious magical types. We exchanged a few emails and agreed to meet at a restaurant. This was a huge mistake and we will cover why later.

When I arrived at the restaurant, I noticed a guy walking parallel to me glance over and smile. This guy couldn't possibly be him. I ignored him as I entered the restaurant and scanned the room for my magician. As luck would have it, parking lot guy walked over, introduced himself, and asked if I was Cathy. This David Copperfield had aged about 20 years since his modeling picture, had a receding hairline, and a huge comb-over to combat it. I am not a shallow girl but this guy clearly misrepresented himself online.

He asked me to sit for dinner and I reluctantly agreed. I was totally unprepared for this scenario. I was in an awkward position but instead of leaving, I felt embarrassed and stayed. I kept asking myself what I could order to make this date quick. To make matters even more uncomfortable, every time someone opened the door to the restaurant, a woosh of wind would whip his comb-over up and it would wave at me. I didn't know whether to giggle or give it a high-five. Awkward!

My nightmare date had one really endearing quality – he couldn't stop talking about how cool he was and how much money he made. He would end his statements with a proud snort and giggle. Ugh. It was the longest dinner ever! When we finished, I insisted on paying for my own meal, excused myself, and left. When I got to my car, reality hit. I just put myself in a bad situation with a man I didn't know, who could have harmed me. He misrepresented himself online, and who knows what else he could have lied about. Has this happened to you?

A great way to avoid this situation is to remember that, although he may look adorable in his pictures and seem disarmingly witty in the emails, it could all be a total fake, so keep your guard up. You might want to ask him for several pictures to compare. I'm not saying to ask for the one that's like a hostage forced to take a picture holding a newspaper as proof of what he really looks like, but a few recent candid shots should give you an accurate view.

The Email Inquisition

Let email be your first way of communicating with a would-be date. When I was dating online, I set up a secondary email for the service, so I wouldn't have to give out my personal email. That way I didn't have to worry about sifting through the emails from the dating site to get to my personal emails. You also avoid a whole lot of spam emails going to your personal account. I got tons when I subscribed to the dating site.

Email lets you chat with complete anonymity. When someone seems interesting, have a marathon email session with him. Take your time to discover your compatibility. Ask the hard questions. Do some research on what he is telling you about himself and his experiences. Practice being fearless and take charge. Because you are Internet savvy, it is easy to look him up online. If he is on a social networking site, then go on and read his posts; read the "about me" section, and look at his pictures. Be your own detective and cover all your bases. If he passes your little investigation, his online information looks decent, and he really takes time to open up, he may be worth your time to get to know.

Bear in mind if something doesn't seem right or you decide he is not the one for you, then politely tell him you're not interested. If he doesn't take the hint then just block his emails. It's a lot easier and cheaper to block emails or just stop using a secondary email you set up than to change your phone number and contact everyone you know to give them your new number because some creepy guy can't take a hint. Be resourceful!

The Meet and Greet

Okay, let's say he passes the email stage and you decide you'd like to meet him in person. I strongly recommend meeting him first before giving him your number. Let's assume you do give him your number and chat with him a bit before making your date. His voice on the phone is so dreamy, you start to wonder what could possibly go wrong? The answer is, lots, and a Fabulous girl like you shouldn't take chances. Remember back at the restaurant with my strange magician? It's a great idea to set up what I like to call the "Meet and Greet". It is your plan A escape. The Meet and Greet is usually held at a coffee house or ice cream shop a distance from your home. (You don't want your jilted Mr. Creepy following you home if you have to ditch him.) These kinds of places offer you a sweet getaway if you show up and your Mr. Dreamy is actually a creep. Have a cup of coffee, keep the conversation light because you have manners, and then you are out! In a half hour to an hour, tops, you are ready to sashay your way out the door and on to your next adventure. How's that for awesome?

Pay attention to your surroundings as you leave, go straight to your car, get in, and go. You could text your friends about the date later from home. Your objective at the moment is to get out of there. You really don't know this person and he may have dark intentions, so the quicker you leave, the sooner you can forget this date ever happened.

But if he turns out to be awesome, then your cup of coffee can turn into great conversation, dinner, and dancing. Call a friend and let her know what is happening, and send her the picture you cunningly took before you head out. Remember, Fearless, even though you think he is charming, you don't know him yet, so you drive yourself to your next destination. If the night turns out to be a flop, you could always jump in your car and drive away.

At the end of the night, even if your date is magical, you still mind your manners and make him wait to actually know the real you by saying your goodnights, getting in your car, and going home. I promise you will leave his mind wandering and heart racing. No one makes the VIP list to get into your home easily, especially on the first date. You are Fabulous and worth the wait.

Social Media Confidential

Social media can be so intoxicatingly addictive. You could be sitting in the comfort of your home, office, school, or library and chatting with people from exotic places around the world or right down the street — all at the tips of your fingers. You share your views and read the feelings of others. Everything is instantaneous. Thoughts, statements, jokes, and ideas are constantly flowing. It's so easy to get carried away in the rush of information being exchanged. You belong to groups and circles in your online social scene. You have fans, friends, and followers, some of whom you have never met before, reading all about you. Honestly, the reach is amazing.

Life is an open book in social media. It is as open as

you allow it to be. It seems as though we are getting to a point where nothing is secret anymore. You share so much of your life through your stories and pictures with friends as well as complete strangers. Everyone is posting pictures of themselves, their homes, kids, friends, and offices. We post what we are doing, wearing, and where we are going several times a day.

We also tend to get competitive when it comes to social media — competitive as in who has more followers and friends online, and who is doing something more exciting than anyone else. We find ourselves trying to do the next best thing to get those compliments, responses, RTs, and follows we need to make us feel good and important. We have all been sucked into that fame game. Be cautious, Fearless. The Internet is filled with trolls and monsters. Your innocent post about going to the local theater along with the snap shot of what you are wearing before you leave can be an invitation to danger.

Jenn Gibbs is a pretty Fabulous woman. She decided she was not going to stand on the sidelines and just feel helpless when it comes to raising awareness about breast cancer. She stepped up to do something. And by something, I don't mean a little something. She rowed the 1,500 mile perimeter of Lake Michigan, ending her journey in Chicago. She did it because she is amazing and because one of her "likes" is kicking cancer's butt! You go girl!

What a great cause. On her website, Row4Row.org, Jenn was keeping up with her supporters by posting in a daily online journal, sharing her exact location so eager fans and well-wishers could keep track of her progress. Unbeknownst to her, there was a monster tracking her as well.

Early Sunday morning on July 22, while Jenn was docked in a remote area of the lake, a man entered Jenn's boat cabin, attacked, and sexually assaulted her. The police believe this man drove a considerable distance just to attack her.

"I still believe that there are more good people in the world than bad. I still believe that life is a gift, even when it's scary and unfair. I still believe that life offers us the privilege, the opportunity, and the responsibility, to give something back, even when people try to take things away from us."

Jenn Gibbons

Jenn is a fighter, though! A couple of days after this terrible ordeal, she showed incredible bravery, determination, and grace. She got right back into her journey and completed her mission.

I have met criminals who were convinced their victims were actually inviting them along with such naive information. The sick mind of a monster could twist even the most innocent statements, so be aware.

Realize that the Internet remembers everything. There are data bases that collect all sorts of information, and a search of your name will usually bring up a surprising amount of information you didn't know was available. I recommend, if you are going to get heavily involved with social networking for fun, posting anonymously. Don't use your real name. Use a nickname to identify yourself. If you are going to use your real name, turn on your privacy settings to limit who can view your information and updates. Make vague statements of where you are going and what you are currently doing. Or, if you are really excited about your adventure, post the information after the fact. After you are home safe, you could then relive your escapades with a blog post or update to share with your many friends.

Imagine this happening to you. You are home alone in your apartment in the city. You live alone (well actually, not totally alone, but in the company of your dog). You have your daily routines like walking your dog twice a day, going to work in the morning, going to work out, etc. You also have an online journal or blog. One night, you get an email from a stranger. He asks you some odd questions, personal questions that he would know only if he was watching you. He tells you what your routine is and what you are doing in the privacy of your home. You ignore him but he sends you another few emails with even more details about your activities.

It is now very obvious he is spying on you, but how? He reveals to you information you have posted online. A quick search on your end pops up a wealth of information about you that you inadvertently shared and didn't know was so easily accessible. He has pictures of you, your dog, and who knows what else. Something like this happened to a girl online. The guy had perhaps seen her, then followed her to her apartment building and observed her for a while, possibly finding her name on the mail box and searching her name online. He spooked her to the point that the only way she could feel safe again was to get away from that place, find another apartment, and be more careful about her information exchange and privacy settings.

Do a search of your name and see what comes up. If you feel the information is personal, click on the link and find the source to delete it. Often we could go back and find the original post we made and delete it.

Picture Perfect

You love having lots of people in your network to share your experience. It is easy to get swept up into doing whatever it takes to expand your circle. We become experts in the art of the self-portrait or mirror shot. The peace sign with duck lip pose. Perhaps a naughty or risqué shot every once in a while. This is especially true with young girls.

Break yourself of this habit. You are a classy girl who doesn't need to reduce herself to a mirror shot for compliments in order to feel good. Your lips look better with a smile than with the puckered duck look. Never post a sexy or compromising picture of yourself. So many of us have impulsively posted things we regret later. One reckless post or picture on the Internet, one lapse of judgment, and that picture could come back to haunt you later. This is a trail already blazed with warning signs all over it. Don't do it.

Many a monster can now copy and save your pictures from your social site, rather than stalking you, to take your picture in person. The Internet makes it so much easier for a pervert to pursue you and follow your every move. Think before you do anything careless. Carefully consider the information being shared with strangers. Use a nickname, but if you choose to use your real name, then protect yourself with your privacy settings. Properly set controls keep the unwanted creepers out of your site and your pictures protected. All social sites have them. Once your private picture is out there, it is virtually impossible to get it erased completely off the Internet. The Internet never forgets. If you practice thinking strategically long enough, it will become a habit.

Even If you really, really like him and think this may be your future husband, don't do it! He is a stranger. You are a wonderful woman who is worth the wait. Too much too soon rarely gets the Prince. Once you are alone with a stranger, the unthinkable can happen.

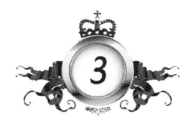

The life of the Party!

Partying

A Fabulous girl like you knows how to have a good time and has lots of friends to join you. Mixing and mingling is your specialty. You and your girls love to dance and party. Your party ritual starts at home before you go out. You blast music while getting ready to rock it with the girls. You prepare for the night by getting dressed, make-up on, hair done, and by putting together your nightclub "must haves". Your "must haves" are your ID, purse, money, keys, charged cell phone, and lipstick. Later I will have some safety "must haves" recommendations for you to consider when you are going out.

Once ready, you head out in your most stylish outfit. You are in pink alert mode, and ready to have a good time. You know what places you're going to hit, where to meet if you get separated, and who will be the non-drinking D.D. (Designated Driver).

When you arrive at the club, you valet park when you can, or park in the closest spot possible. If you are in a garage, you park closest to the elevator or a brightly lit spot. No one wants to walk too far in stilettos, so convenience is a little bonus to safety. Scan the area as you are looking for a good spot to park. Stay away from loiterers or, if something looks suspect, just keep driving. It is better to be safe than sorry. Don't linger in the car when you park. You might inadvertently attract unwanted attention from someone looking for an easy target. When you sit in your car after you park, you give someone looking to do something a chance to set up for an attack. They have a chance to see if you are alone, how many people are with you, and if you have a guy with you or are just with girls. If you are not quick moving, they have the upper hand in the surprise. When you park, take a second to scan the immediate area right outside your car, and once clear, get out right away. You are more likely to see someone slinking around or standing outside your car rather than with the limited view you have sandwiched between two cars. With a quick exit from your car, a creep usually won't have the chance to crouch down and surprise you.

Never leave anything of value visible in the car. You don't want to return later to find your window smashed and car ransacked. There is nothing worse than coming back to your car after a fun night out and dealing with the shock of having your car broken into. Ugh. I'm telling you from firsthand experience; it could take your night from fun to downer very quickly.

Now it's time to have fun. You are the queen on the scene, in control, and anyone who sees you knows it. You are confident and aware. Your demeanor says you are here to have a good time but will not hesitate to kick butt if the need to protect yourself arises. Throughout my years interviewing and studying criminals, the one constant was the opportunity of the crime. The victim usually was a weak-looking easy target. Not you! Girl, you exude beauty, focus, awareness, and bravery.

Follow these tips and you won't go wrong:

- Bring your friends.
- Valet park.
- Park close to the venue.
- Have at least one non-drinking friend with you.
- Don't leave your drink alone.
- Never leave with a stranger.
- Be confident.
- Have fun.

A fun attitude and confidence is everything when you are enjoying a night out with friends. Being the smart girl you are, you also have a Fabulous friend who doesn't drink by your side. It is always a good idea to have a friend who doesn't drink because your D.D. could slip if you are having fun and end up drinking, too.

Your sober fabulous girlfriend will also be the one who will step in to shoo away those pesky drunk guys who can get annoying or touchy-feely if you have had a little too much to drink and your judgment is clouded. She will also be your eyes and ears when you have had one too many of those wonderful Cosmos.

"Never violate the sacredness of your individual self respect"

Theodore Parker

You like to have a drink or two but realize that a good time doesn't require you to be drunk and sloppy. You wouldn't be caught dead embarrassing yourself in such a way. You realize that good judgment diminishes when you are drunk. You are not the kind of girl who lets yourself engage in behavior you will regret later. Stumbling around drunk isn't very fun at all.

Hey there Delilah!

This reminds me of a night out with my friend Delilah: One night, while at a club together, Delilah was enjoying her favorite drink – Lifesavers. Actually, she had one too many of her favorite drink and was pretty drunk, but I was there to watch over her and keep her out of trouble. Thinking back on that night, it was pretty embarrassing for both of us. We went to this club often and knew lots of people there. Delilah was acting quite unFabulous with her loud screeching laugh and stumbling walk. In the midst of the drunken chaos she met a guy named Mike and immediately began foolishly fawning over him. We were all chatting and dancing when she suddenly left the dance floor, heading straight to the bathroom. Mike followed her to make sure she was alright. I stayed behind dancing.

Delilah was pretty nauseous and headed to a

stall to throw up. When she was done, she managed to clean herself up and stumble back out to the bar area. Her eye-makeup was running, her hair was tousled, and her lipstick was smeared. Her clothes were disheveled and dotted with puke stains. Mike was waiting for her by the bar closest to the restroom door, swooped her up, and kissed her passionately while getting real handsy with her. Ewwww! He then complimented her on her fruity breath and left when he noticed me charging over. She stood there confused and heaving because even she realized it was gross. Poor Delilah looked a mess. I decided to call it a night and get her home before anyone else noticed her sloppy behavior.

So many things were wrong with that scenario:

- First...GROSS!!! She just threw up and he kissed her... YUCK!

- I was a terrible friend. I should have gone to the bathroom with her because I knew how drunk she was. I was sober and should have known better.

- If Mike had decided to take her, she would have possibly left willingly because of her intoxicated state.

- He could have also possibly taken her by force and she would have been physically unable to make the right choices to keep herself safe.

- She could have fallen and hurt herself.

- She could have wandered off.

Be sharp, Doll. Don't let yourself get carried away by the lure of excess when you are drinking.

You could regret it later. Understand this: you can have a great time without ever taking a drink. Don't feel pressured to drink because others are doing it. Flex your control muscles and determine what is best for you. Do it in even the most minor decisions. Start practicing taking control of your situation with the small stuff, so by the time the major decisions have to be made, you can react in a split second. Always act as if what you decide matters, because it does.

Roofies

While out having cocktails, you should never leave your drink unattended. Drugs such as Roofies and GHB could be slipped into your drink. These drugs are colorless and tasteless and will incapacitate you within minutes. If someone you just met offers you a drink, have him order it in your presence, and take it directly from the bartender or waitress. If you are sitting at a table, and the waitress is busy, and he offers to go to the bar to get it, go with him. If not, decline until the waitress comes around again. Don't take chances.

If you happen to take a drink and start to feel weird or woozy, get help immediately. If you have a friend nearby, go to them for assistance. If no friend is immediately around, then ask a waitress, bartender, or security for help. Tell them you think you have been drugged and don't let anyone take you anywhere except your girlfriend. Point out the guy who gave you the drink to the waitress, bartender, or security so he doesn't get a chance to take you in case you do pass out. You will only have a few minutes before you black out. Blacking out while drugged could mean you could pass out or just not be aware or what is happening or remember anything afterwards. The events will be a blur.

You are classy, so your girlfriends know you wouldn't just leave with a guy. They will always step in to make your decisions for you if you look like you are not acting like yourself. This is what girlfriends do for each other. You always surround yourself with real girlfriends. Girls who are like your sisters — supportive and awesome!

Keep the mystery alive

You are relaxed meeting new people and being social, so when you do meet a cool, handsome new guy you feel comfortable spending some time with, you still remember, even if you are one hundred percent sober, never ever leave with a stranger. If your ride leaves you stranded or your car won't start, just call a cab. Even If you really, really like him and think this may be your future husband, don't do it! He is a stranger. You are a wonderful woman who is worth the wait. Too much too soon rarely gets the Prince. Once you are alone with a stranger, the unthinkable can happen. You are readjusting your life to fearlessly Fabulous and will no longer take chances on being damaged by a monster.

When it gets crazy ...

Bars, nightclubs, parties, and festivals have one thing in common – the later it gets, the crazier people behave. The later the evening gets and the longer people have been drinking, the greater the possibility for problems to occur. Aside from being tacky, standing around when the music stops and the lights come on can be dangerous. There are a lot of very drunk people hanging around. Drunk men have a tendency of getting fresh and potentially violent if rejected. Driving very late at night after a club has closed increases the likelihood of encountering drunk drivers out on the road.

Another issue to address is the "liquid courage" that shows up after a few too many drinks. After several hours of drinking, just one wrong look could send fists and bottles flying. People who are drunk don't always behave, and if you are there you could get caught up in the fray. If you notice that something doesn't look right or there is a commotion, move in the other direction. Get away. Getting hit on the face by a flying bottle isn't very fun. It always amazes me to see people running to see a fight happening. If they were going to stop the fight, I could respect that, but they usually want to get a front row spot to watch or record someone pummeling another. That can come with consequences like a punch in the face and a trip to the hospital because you got swept up in the melee and got hurt. You are smarter than that — you just go!

Leaving doesn't mean your night has to end. My friends and I would leave a club and head out to an all-night diner or pizza parlor. It was the best. We would grab a bite, unwind, and laugh about the fun night we'd just had. Sometimes we would bump into people from the club and just hang out without all the noise and strobe lights to just chat. A lot of times that was my favorite part of the night.

A Fabulous night out with friends should end with you sweating from dancing hard, feet sore because you mingled the whole night, and cheeks hurting because you spent the evening smiling and laughing! The next morning you should wake up with a clear memory and stories to share with your girls.

"A much more effective and lasting method of facelifting than surgical technique is happy thinking, new interests, and outdoor exercise"

– Dr. Sara Murray Jordan

Zen Fabulous

Jogging, hiking, and outdoor activities

What could be more relaxing than taking a nice hike in your favorite neighborhood park or scenic wooded area? Keeping Fabulously fit and in shape is what you are about. There is nothing like getting outdoors and feeling the sun on your face and wind in your hair. Although it seems as if this should be a sanctuary, it is not. Danger could be anywhere. A Fearless girl will always take a friend with her. What could be better than a relaxing scenic jog with your bestie? Being safe while you have fun.

Jogging

When heading out for an outdoor activity like jogging, keep some simple tips in mind. Don't go out late at night or in the early morning alone. If the only time you can go out is at those times, then do it someplace where there are lots of people around. Go to a local track where there are other runners. Get a running buddy. Join a running club. You are sure to have plenty of running buddies when you are part of a group. There is safety in numbers as well as a great time. How amazing to be able to do something you enjoy with friends who like it too! Some items you should always have with you are a great pair of running shoes, water, cell phone, and a small metal object you could use to defend yourself if the need arises.

Nicole Ganguzza was a vibrant 26-year-old newlywed from New Jersey living in Orlando, Florida, with her new husband. The couple were avid outdoorsmen who enjoyed cycling and running together. Back in high school Nicole was captain of her cross-country team and used to run to relax. On the early evening of June 10, 2008, Nicole called her husband to tell him she was going for a run on a new trail they had discovered earlier while cycling together. He never heard from her again. The next day her body was found approximately 50 feet off the trail, half covered with bushes.

Shortly after Nicole's attack, a woman walking her dog alone in the same park was attacked, pulled into the woods, and had her shirt ripped open in an attempted rape. She managed to get away, screaming for help. Then, a few days later, another woman who had stopped riding her bike to get a drink of water, was dragged into the woods. Luckily, she too managed to escape. It happens. Attacks like these don't always make the national news, but they do happen and a lot more often than we care to acknowledge.

In the Zone

Remember listening to music while jogging can be exhilarating and help you get in the zone, but never have the music in your headphones playing so loud that you cannot hear what is going on around you. Blasting your favorite songs can sure amp up your running experience, but it can disable your ability to maintain awareness of your surroundings. You are in complete white alert mode when you tune out of the real world and sink into your running zone. If you are attacked, you will be completely caught off guard and disoriented. Enjoy your moment, but keep in mind your safety above all else.

A Fearless girl is always prepared to take whatever steps are necessary to stop an aggressor from hurting her and to get away. She always remembers these four things:

- ✓ Bring the right equipment.
- ✓ Don't disable your sense of awareness.
- ✓ Bring a friend.
- ✓ Have a plan.

Biking

Riding your bike is such great exercise! It's a wonderful way to get around and stay in shape. Please be smart about it, Girl. Keep in mind that, although it is a useful and green way to travel, it is not always safe. If you find yourself out late one night at a friend's house, do not ride home alone. No matter how close your home is, it is unsafe to do so. Monsters use the cloak of darkness to look for easy prey. You have little chance of being seen or helped if you are alone at night riding a bike and are attacked.

Let us remember the story of Michaela "Mickey" Shunick. She was a college student who loved riding her bike. One Friday night she decided to ride home from a friend's house at close to 2 a.m. She lived a short distance away and thought it was a good idea. She had made these treks many times before. On this night she never made it home. The next day she missed her brother's graduation and the following Monday her birthday. She would have been 22. A huge effort was mounted by her family, friends, and strangers to find her. Police turned up a couple grainy surveillance pictures showing her riding in the street on the route she always took to go home. The surveillance tapes also caught a couple vehicles on the same street she was riding, and, by process of elimination, as they identified the vehicles, they determined that the likely suspect vehicle was a white truck.

A week later, her damaged bike was spotted by two fishermen under a bridge 27 miles away from where she was spotted on surveillance.

A couple months later, a convicted sexual predator was arrested and charged with her murder. This monster was convicted in 2000 for sexual battery and was released in 2008. The police say the evening Mickey went missing, the predator was driving around, [they believe] looking for someone vulnerable to victimize. Mickey rolled onto the mostly empty street and the opportunity presented itself to him.

Mickey's body was found shortly after his arrest, buried in a shallow grave just beyond a small cemetery in the woods.

As we go on, let us think about what could have been done differently to prevent such a tragedy from happening again. Riding your bike at night alone comes with risks. I would love to say you are safe, but the truth is, you are not. Monsters such as this predator love the low visibility of night to find their victims. At night there is the likelihood that a beast could escape. There are fewer prying eyes at night and that is exactly what a criminal is counting on. At night you are more likely to be in an impaired state, whether by exhaustion or intoxication, making you an easier target.

We tell ourselves that we will not live in fear and that we will do what we want because we won't let fear overcome us. You should learn to embrace fear in order to protect yourself. You need to think about potential threats in order to not become a victim. Being fearless means that you know fear, can identify a threat, and do what it takes to be safe. As a result, you "fear less."

Don't allow yourself to be someone's victim. Be smart in your decisions and safety. Looking back at Mickey's scenario, just one decision could have changed the whole situation. Had she just asked her friend for a ride home instead of riding her bike alone, things would have turned out differently. She would have been there beaming with pride on Saturday morning at her brother's graduation and on Monday she would have celebrated her 22nd birthday with family and the same friends who desperately searched for her.

If not for that one decision, we would not have known her name or seen her innocent face on the news, and that would have been fine. It would have meant that she was busy going on with her life — instead of becoming a life now cut short, and creating a family left searching for answers, friends left wondering why, and broken hearts.

So many things can go wrong, and you need to adjust your behavior and think ahead of all the possibilities. Being out alone on the street at night exposes you to so many unnecessary risks. You could be kidnapped.

You could get hit by a driver who doesn't see you on the road in the dark. You could be struck by a drunk driver. You could fall and hurt yourself and perhaps not be found until the next morning. You could get a flat and have to walk while dragging a bike with you. Why take chances? Get a ride home and come back for your bike in the morning. Taking precautions is not living in fear — it's learning to live "fear less."

Hiking

Hiking is fantastic. It is a way of connecting with nature and all its beauty. There are some of the most beautiful places to hike right here in the U.S. as well as around the world. It is peaceful and a way to escape the everyday routine as well as the noise of the city. Doesn't that sound wonderful? Every girl needs an escape sometimes to relax and reconnect with herself.

There are lots of things to keep in mind when out on a nature adventure:

- ✓ Take proper equipment.
- ✓ Wear good shoes.
- ✓ Nature is unpredictable, so be prepared to turn back .
- ✓ Don't do it alone. There is a risk for injury and a lone hiker may not be able to call for help.
- ✓ Know how to rescue yourself.
- ✓ Enjoy

When taking a hike, long or short, the best advice is to always be prepared. Having the proper equipment will ensure a wonderful experience. Always bring along water, a map, compass, cell phone (although some hiking routes may not have cell reception), snacks, whistle, rain gear, flashlight, first aid kit, and a weapon of some sort. Whether that weapon is mace, a gun, a knife, or baton, bring something. Along with those items also have a good pair of hiking shoes and the right clothing for the seasonal weather.

Mother Nature is awesome but she can be moody. One minute it can be bright and shiny and the next there are rainstorms, windstorms, or snowstorms. Being properly clothed will keep you ahead of any little twist in the weather thrown your way. Be mindful that even if it is an unseasonably warm or hot day, the temperatures on high hills or mountains could be much different, so be prepared.

Hiking up beautiful nature trails and getting lost in the breath-taking scenery is the reason it is so popular, but keep in mind there are also animals out on the trails. If you don't pay attention, you could be on the wrong side of the trail between a mama bear and her cubs and find yourself in a whole lot of trouble. That is when a calm demeanor and mace could be your friend. Although the best advice I could give you is to just be aware and try to avoid this situation altogether; sometimes it is impossible. If you encounter a bear on your hike, try to remain calm and quietly back away. Speak in a monotone, calm voice, and wave your arms so the bear can identify you as human and not prey. In some cases, if there is a good distance between you and the bear, you could try to climb a tall tree. If the bear is within 25 feet of you and is closing in, mace him. Whatever you do, just don't run! A bear can chase you down on any terrain. This is their land and this is what they do. Just try to remain calm. Before heading out, research bear activity and response preparedness on the park website. Being informed is the best way to make your hike safe and fun.

The truly best way to hike is with a group of people. Once you start out, always stay with the group and end with the group. If you want to venture out, tell the group which trail you will hike, when you will return, and your emergency plan. Always have one of those. If you want a bit of solitude to meditate, it is best if you still go with at least one friend. Actually, if that is what you want, then pick a friend who is experienced with the outdoors. The outdoors can be tricky and dangerous.

Know how to read your map and compass. Stay on your trail. If you want to venture off the trail to explore a cave or a pretty ridge, keep your trail tagged or within view at all times. If an emergency occurs, you may get disoriented and lose sight of the trail and get lost. If you do happen to get lost, stop and study your map. Look around to reorient yourself with your surroundings. You may need to get to a higher vantage point to identify landmarks. If you are still lost, then grab your whistle and blow it at regular intervals to attract attention. Keep it safe by staying with a group.

Monster on the trail

Be keenly aware that animals of the hairy variety are not the only things to look out for in the mountains or woods. There are some sick people who use these iso-lated areas to find victims to attack. For this reason, I urge you to never go at it alone. Even with a group, keep your eyes and ears open just like you would for a bear. And always have your weapon ready for action.

The outdoors is amazing, and getting out of your

house, school, or office to enjoy it is an absolute must for every Fabulous girl! Get into your comfy clothes, close your books, turn off your computer and get out there!

"Keep your face to the sunshine" – Helen Keller

You are secure, alert, and won't be an easy mark. A criminal is looking for an easy victim. He knows that with your self-confidence and awareness you won't be easy to attack. There is no element of surprise with you, and you are shining a light on him.

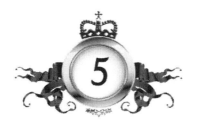

Retail Therapy Shopping

Shopping is a sacred event for every Fabulous girl. You hit the stores with the energy and intensity of an Olympian. You know your favorite stores, the latest styles, and where the best deals are happening. You are on pink alert while you breeze around from shop to shop. Your hands are filled with bags of the latest styles but you keep your eyes and ears alert to the people around you.

Be F.A.B.
Focused
Aware
Brave

One evening a couple years ago, I was having a little retail therapy session at a mall a few blocks away from my home. When I arrived, I noticed a man staring at me but paid no attention. I noticed this same man again as I was walking out of a store. This time I paid attention. He made me uncomfortable. My alert level now rose to orange; I remained calm and tried to continue shopping in hopes I was mistaken and seeing him twice staring at me was just a coincidence. I headed into a store to look at the clothes, but at this point I was just testing him to see what he would do next.

He followed me into the shop and stood at one of the racks with his elbow up on the bar, leaning forward towards me, and asked my name. I told him to leave me alone and left the store. He followed behind me as I walked through the mall, occasionally stopping to pretend to look at something if I turned to see where he was. I was starting to panic, but I knew as long as I stayed in this busy place until I could formulate an exit plan, I was safe.

I walked the mall a couple times thinking of what to do. I noticed 2 police officers walking through the exit where I was parked. One of them happened to be an acquaintance. Perfect. (Every girl should have at least one police friend.) I approached them and told them about what was happening. I described the guy who was following me without looking back, so he wouldn't know what I was doing. I then walked passed them and through the exit. Mr. Creepy jumped up and started after me. My buddy then stepped in front of him to talk, to delay him just long enough for me to get to my car and go. As I was driving away, I watched him run out of the mall and scan the parking lot before turning and going back inside. Scary!

This event ended safely because I didn't dismiss my intuitions. I felt like something was wrong and made a plan to get away safely. Trust your instinct. Don't dismiss your gut feeling. If someone at a mall, store, theater, or anywhere else is making you uncomfortable, get away from the area or seek help. There are literally dozens of creepy people lurking around malls and other places of entertainment, waiting for their opportunity to strike. Always know your exits. You are fierce, smart, and ready. You know they are there and how to stay one step ahead of them.

You are secure, alert, and won't be an easy mark. A criminal is looking for an easy victim. He knows that with your self-confidence and awareness you won't be easy to attack. There is no element of surprise with you, and you are shining a light on him. This is YOUR second sanctuary and you know how to work it.

- Be on Pink Alert.
- Keep your purse closed.
- Don't flaunt your valuables.
- Look around.
- Know your exits.
- Go Go Go

Always trust your instincts. Most people are in white alert mode while shopping, more so than in any other place, because there are sales and the latest designs to see. And, after you shop, you are typically thinking about the outfits you bought, where you will wear them, and how fierce you are going to look. Snap out of it!

Plastic makes perfect

You pay for your cool new items with a card. Paying in cash is so yesterday. If you pull out a wad of cash from your purse to count it at checkout you are only bringing unnecessary attention to yourself. A thief doesn't know you only have $40 in your purse. He only sees you have cash. Cash is quick and liquid. It is easier for him to take your cash to use than your credit card, which could possibly get him caught.

Remember to close your purse after every purchase. It may seem logical but you would be surprised how many times you toss your wallet back in, grab your bags, and forget to close your purse. Who could blame you? You just got some amazing new clothes at a great deal and you're excited. Take a few extra seconds to make sure everything is secure before you walk away from the register.

When shopping at a jewelry store, ask them to place your items in an unmarked bag. If they don't have unmarked bags, then place the item in another one of your shopping bags or your purse.

My 78 year old mother went to pick up jewelry cleaning solution at a jewelry store. When she left the store with her little bag that said the name on it, two thieves pushed her down and took her bag from her. Luckily, she wasn't too terribly hurt, although she was pretty shaken up. It goes to show the reality that criminals are willing to take their chances if they even see a potential of stealing something valuable. Don't give them that chance.

Know your exits.

Know exactly where your exit points are at all times. If something happens, you get out of there immediately. Don't look back, and don't head towards the problem to see what is going on. Just go. Better to be safe than sorry and, unless you are a secret super hero, there is nothing you can do other than call the police as you get to safety.

Once you are done shopping, scan your surroundings and be aware of anyone who may be following you. Before you leave the store, have your keys in your hand with the car key between your index and middle finger or your kubotan (we'll cover what this is later) in hand. Anyone thinking of doing you harm is in for a rude awakening. You head straight for your car while scanning the surrounding area. You always have one arm free of bags. It just makes it much easier to react to a problem if you have a free hand. Once in your car, lock the door, turn on your car, and go. The most dangerous time while out shopping is the walk from your car to the store and from the store to your car. Now is not the time to fuss with your bags, fix your makeup, talk on the phone, or text. Get the car moving and out of the spot. Once you are out, you can then pull over at an outdoor parking lot to compose that text message or fix your makeup. Moving objects aren't easy to hit, so the quicker you leave the parking spot you were in, the better.

Following these safety tips will ensure you fully enjoy every shopping trip. You have more important things to think about than worrying about your stolen purse or goodie bag that was lost to some thief who took advantage of you because you were not paying attention. You are becoming a Fearlessly alert girl. Nothing takes you by surprise anymore. By being keenly aware of things going on around you, you are taking control.

"You educate a man; you educate a man. You educate a woman; you educate a generation."

–Brigham Young

Higher Learning and Other Fun Stuff!

College Safety

College is one of the most excellent experiences of a Fabulous girl's life. It is your first taste of freedom. You have complete control over the direction of your life for the first time. This is the place where all the possibilities of your life will start to materialize. You are going to have a Fabulous future and it will start here.

Just as there are possibilities for positive changes, so are there possibilities for bad things to happen. You have to always be on pink alert. Be aware of your surroundings at all times. If you have a late class in the evening that requires you to walk through buildings and parking lots to get to class, try to have a classmate with you. Make friends with your classmates. Join study groups. In other words, surround yourself with people. The more people you know, the better. There are two benefits to that. First, you will make new friends and possible life-long companions, and second, you will make great contacts for networking.

All campuses have escort services, but if somehow you find yourself alone, be vigilant and walk with purpose. Keep one arm free at all times. Have your keys in hand, walk along well-lit areas, and go straight to your car or dorm. If something or someone raises your level of alert to orange, find a safe place to go, like a bookstore, or a group of people to talk to until the threat moves on, or ask for someone to walk you to safety. Familiarize yourself with the emergency phones located all around campus.

Campus Living

Living on campus is a blast. This is your first taste of what living in the real world is like, within a safe environment, with one exception; all your neighbors are your friends and close in age. How sweet is that? You have a few choices of where to live - there are the residence halls, sorority houses, and off-campus housing.

Residence halls are usually divided up into women-only and men-only wings, or sometimes the whole building is designated male or female. They are located right on campus, so getting around is quite convenient. Halls are generally secure, usually requiring keys or pass codes to get into the building. Living here gives you convenience, your own private spot, and freedom.

Sororities are social clubs for women enrolled in college. They're all-girls clubs that offer great places to live and be social with other Fabulous girls. Actually, the others in your sorority are called your "sisters". Your sisters will be a great support during your time in school and long after. You can never have too many besties and sisters.

"Act as if what you do makes a difference. It does."

William James

For the more independent spirit, there is plenty of off-campus housing available. The one drawback I find with that arrangement is that you are slightly more isolated and out of touch with the others who live on campus. If you can, it is best to apply early to get your housing on campus, so you can be close to the action and fun.

Parties and Games

College is also a time for some pretty amazing events and parties. These parties and events will be fueled by lots of adrenaline and alcohol. Enjoy every second of the college experience, but remember a few tips to keeping yourself safe:

- Know your limits.
- Keep a friend who doesn't drink with you.
- Stay away from drugs.
- Keep your drink in your possession at all times and, if possible, serve it yourself.
- Try to only drink from a bottle you opened.
- If something feels wrong, get away.
- If you start to feel physically impaired even if you didn't have that many drinks, alert a sober friend or call a friend to pick you up immediately. If you have been drugged, you will only have a few minutes before you pass out.
- Do not leave with someone you don't know.
- Don't shut the party down. The longer you stay,

the drunker others will be and the more possibility there will be for trouble to happen.

↙ Follow your intuition.

↙ Never buckle to peer pressure.

You are smart and savvy. You know yourself better than anyone. You know your limits with alcohol; you have boundaries, and would never cross them. There is a threshold between tipsy and slushy. Everyone's line is different. I don't drink. I just don't enjoy the fact that I get sick very quickly. I go from tipsy to sloppy in 2.0 beers. Others can drink quite a bit and still be pretty composed and functional. You know what your limits are. I'm a total lightweight, so I just decided that it is not for me. I am also the first one up on stage singing with the band and dancing wildly. If you don't drink, don't be afraid to speak up and decline a drink. If you are feeling a bit of pressure from others, just volunteer to be the designated driver. Show them you don't need to drink to have a good time. If you are underage, just pass up drinking altogether. All schools have zero tolerance for underage drinking and so do the police. Why risk it?

"It is better to displease the people by doing what is right, than to temporarily please them by doing what you know is wrong."

William Boetcker

If you do drink, then it is a good idea to have a friend who doesn't drink with you. Unlike a club, college parties have lots of free or cheap drinks, so out-of-control drinking is easy. Your nondrinking friend will be your alert eyes and ears as well as your safe ride home or escort to your dorm.

One night, at one of the famed frat parties at a big university, Maddie and Laura found themselves doing keggers and drinking excessively. They reached a point where they both admitted they had crossed their limits. Sometimes being in the midst of the party, we allow ourselves to overindulge. Excessive drinking clouds judgment and reasonable thoughts. The next thing they knew, they woke up in their dorm room, naked, and with cigarette burns all over their backs and rear. They both knew that they had been sexually assaulted and were horrified. They most probably had their drinks spiked with a drug. They couldn't remember anything about the evening, and they were humiliated. Maddie told me she remembered snapshots of the night but didn't have a clear picture of the night as a whole. They blanked out and could not remember when or how they ended up getting back to the dorm. They didn't tell the authorities, their parents, or the university out of fear and embarrassment. Maddie left school. Laura finished out the term and transferred to another school.

What an eye opener! Although most parties end innocently enough, there are exceptions. Don't put yourself in a position to be a victim. Remember that sober friend? Had Maddie or Laura been sober, the night might have ended differently. Keep in mind, too, that the later you stay at the party, the drunker others will be, and you place yourself in a prime spot for something negative to happen. Let's be realistic; if someone has bad intent and you are his target, having a clear mind will help you be smart about getting away from the situation.

If you are going to drink at these parties, keep these personal rules in mind – pour your own drink or watch as it's being made, try to drink only from a bottle and maintain control of it at all times (don't put it down and walk away), and if you start to feel weird or impaired, get to a friend immediately! If your drink has been spiked you will only have minutes before you pass out.

These steps could be the difference between waking up after a good, fun night or with cigarette burns and as the victim of a rape.

Don't let yourself be intimidated by peer pressure to drink. When I was in my early twenties, I felt I had to drink to feel like I was having a good time because it was what my friends were doing. It is so unattractive to be a follower. After a few bad hangovers, I decided it was not worth it. I stopped drinking. It was such a relief! I felt better; the morning after felt better; I was in control and loving it. Fabulous, this is your time to shine and have fun! Who has time for a hangover?

When the party is over

Don't shut a party down. What I mean is, don't stay until the last song has played and everyone is lying around in a giant drunken mess. It's so unflattering to be standing around after it is all over. By the end of the night, the level of drunken stupors and testosterone is sky-high and a prime time for some drunk guy to try to get lucky with you. Keep your friends close and never leave with a stranger. It is just not worth exposing yourself to danger. You are Fabulous! A one-night stand is so unFabulous.

Big Games

Home team rallies and games are a blast! You've got a sea of people chanting, cheering, and motivating the team. Everyone is dressed in team colors and there is a palpable excitement in the air.

Before games there are the best pre-game tailgates with barbecues, music, and games while everyone waits for the main event to start. Often there is quite a bit of drinking, so all the earlier rules should apply. Remember, having fun doesn't mean you have to embarrass yourself or end up sick.

Be keenly aware of the group of guys who are getting a little too rowdy and out of control. Steer clear of them. Booze plus adrenaline and testosterone can make for a bad situation. Let the boys get wild while you keep a cool distance. You wouldn't want someone to spill a beer on you and ruin your cute outfit. Above all, remember it's about having fun and keeping safe!

You have a wonderful life ahead of you. Focus on your education, your friends, and (most importantly) yourself. You are going to go far in life. Enjoy this time. What you do now matters, so shine!

Look around the next time you are on a subway train. Do you have a quick getaway when the train stops if you need it? Are you sitting closest to the doors, so you can slip out at the first sign of danger? Do you see anyone who can possibly pose a threat to you as you move through the station?

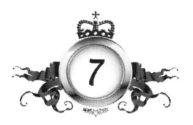

Transportation Whoas

Cars, Subways, and Trains

Cars are crucial to getting around in everyday life for most of us. When we get into our cars, we feel like we are totally safe and secure. We often take for granted that cars could be both our friend and enemy. When you get into your car, the first thing you should do is lock the door. Even before you put on your seat belt, LOCK the door. The last thing a girl wants is a creep sliding into the seat next to her. When out driving late, be mindful of those driving around you. Late at night, others on the road could be intoxicated or driving tired. Both of those are dangerous.

The Fly-By

One night, driving home on the highway with my girl-friends, I noticed a car following us pretty closely on this mostly empty stretch of road. I switched lanes a couple times to see what the driver would do. He followed my moves and maintained a close distance behind me. My alert jumped from pink to orange. I controlled my panic so I could think of a way to get out of the situation safely. Then it hit me – The "Fly-By". I moved over to the far right lane, slowed down to about 15 mph below the speed limit, and waited. The car pulled around to my left (as I had hoped) and we spotted three rowdy guys inside with their windows down, yelling at us. We couldn't understand what they were saying, but they were scaring us. They kept waving and gesturing for us to pull over. I checked my mirrors to see if there was smoke coming out of the back of the car but everything was clear. I didn't feel the familiar thud and wobble of a flat tire, so I decided that continuing to a safe place was the best option, rather than pulling over to see what they wanted from us or stopping to check if anything was wrong with the car.

We said nothing to them, made no eye contact, and just tried to ignore them until we could figure out how we were going to set up the "Fly-By". When they realized we weren't following along they became angry, screaming obscenities at us. I noticed the next familiar exit was a mile ahead. I accelerated back up to the speed limit and the driver did the same to stay right next to me. I inconspicuously used my eyes to look at my rearview mirror, and my girlfriend sitting in the back seat carefully looked for cars to my right, merging onto the highway from the exit lanes. Luckily it was all clear. The guys started waving bottles at us and throwing cups at my car to get me to pull over. As we approached the exit, I abruptly slowed down and exited at the last second, leaving the other car no choice but to drive past the exit, safely carrying out a successful "Fly-By". Awesome!

These guys could have been total saints, but I wasn't going to wait around to find out. Their behavior made us feel uncomfortable. They seemed as if they were drunk or on drugs. Even if they weren't, they acted like complete idiots. Remember, Fabulous, think of yourself and your girlfriends first. Don't jeopardize your safety by even communicating with people acting like that. Find a way to safely get away. Obey the speed limits, be mindful of the cars around you, and try to get out of harm's way. My scenario worked out because we kept our cool and didn't panic. Think of ways you could get away if you were caught in this situation. How would you react?

Subways and Trains

If you live in a big city, then you know traveling the subway is an easy, convenient way to get around. With thousands of people milling through the trains and station at any given time, it is hard to be aware of absolutely everyone around you. Once on the train, it is smart to look around at those people closest to you. Pay attention to their mannerisms and whether or not they are preoccupied with you.

My good friend, Farah, has a pretty intense story about an encounter on a subway train.

"I was sitting in the train reading a book, when a group of people entered the train, and a young man sat two seats over. I could see from the corner of my eye that he was looking at me. When it was my stop, I got off, and noticed that he got off, too. When I got on the next train, there he was again — two seats away. Now I was fully aware. Luckily, the next stop was 'Union Station' where all trains converged, so I had an opportunity to 'lose' him. My plan was to pretend to head towards the Westbound train, and then, halfway down, make a quick 180 back up the stairs (as if I had just realized I was in the wrong

61

direction). That way, I'd know for sure if he was after me or whether it was all just a coincidence. Sure enough, when I did my trick, he did the same move. From then on, I just pretended I was unaware (like you acted in the mall), and walked around until I found a Transit worker. I told her that I was being followed. She asked who it was, so I turned around and pointed at him. He was like three feet behind me. She told both of us to wait there, and radioed the subway patrol. Within one minute, two officers showed up. One man stayed behind with him, while another escorted me to my train.

"From riding the train every day to the exact same stops, I became familiar with my position within the train relative to the nearest exit at my stop. I calculated in my mind which route would require the fewest amount of steps from my seat to the outside world. People just don't think — they get on the first car of the train and sit there, while at their stop, the subway exit is more towards the tenth car, so they end up walking ten car-lengths for nothing, which doesn't make any sense.

The more distance you walk, the more visible you are. I used to walk very fast, almost weaving through the crowd as if in a hurry, even when I wasn't. If a mugger wants a victim, they're not going to go for the quick, alert type — they want a sluggish daydreamer."

Farah is a smart, Fearless woman. She pays attention and understands that in order to avoid being a victim, she needs to think ahead about what could be a potentially bad situation. She is in pink alert mode and acts with purpose.

Look around the next time you are on a subway train. Do you have a quick getaway when the train stops if you need it? Are you sitting closest to the doors, so you can slip out at the first sign of danger? Do you see anyone who can possibly pose a threat to you as you move through the station?

Keep these tips in mind the next time you are traveling on the subway or a train:

- ✔ Keep your valuables secure and hidden – Keep your money and goodies safely tucked away while riding the subway or train. Honestly, you are in a tube with nowhere to go, with a bunch of strangers and some possible monsters just looking around for an opportunity. The time it takes for the train to travel to the next station is time he has to watch you as you pull out your valuables. He has time to think of ways to snatch them from you, possibly hurting you in the process.

- ✔ Pay attention to your surroundings and the people around you – Is there someone staring at you? Are there people arguing and causing a disturbance? Be aware of those closest to you but don't dismiss those outside of your immediate area.

- ✔ Don't jump from car to car unless you feel threatened – It is not recommended for you to jump from car to car. You could slip and hurt or kill yourself. I don't recommend doing this risky maneuver but if you feel that you are in danger, then do what you must to get to safety until the train arrives at the next station.

- ✔ Don't stare at others – Aside from being tacky, staring at others could provoke a confrontation.

People who are mentally unstable will approach you if your eyes meet in a stare. I'm sure there is some clinical explanation for that behavior. All I know is that I have seen it first-hand and have tested it out in my place of work years ago when I worked at a hospital for the criminally insane. Drunks will also engage you if you stare at them. Best if you look around confidently but avoid sitting and staring.

✓ Avoid rush hour – If it's an option, avoid riding the subway or train during rush hour. This is peak time in the stations and hundreds of people are milling around, rushing, pushing, brushing up against you, and touching. Your personal space will be invaded. People you don't know or want to be intimate with will squeeze up against you and have very personal contact with you. It is possible for a monster to use this time to pick-pocket you or possibly sexually assault you by touching you inappropriately.

✓ Avoid routines – If you have to take the same route every day, try to mix it up a bit. Vary the times during which you travel. Walk a little further to another train station. Take a cab. Ride an over-ground bus. Make yourself unpredictable. Unpredictable people are harder to follow.

✓ Minimize unnecessary walking travel distance – Don't take the furthest subway car at the station — the one that leaves you furthest from the exit. Subways smell and the quicker you could get back above ground the better. You wouldn't want to be wearing subway stink on your Fabulous clothes or hair.

Getting caught up in a routine is natural. You do something day in and day out and eventually you do it on autopilot. You drift through your routine mechanically and don't pay attention to the world around you. Break yourself of this. Do things with purpose. Be alert and pay attention. You are Fearless and Fabulous and nothing just happens to you anymore. You are a girl with purpose and confidence!

"There is a stubbornness about me that never can bear to be frightened at the will of others. My courage always rises at every attempt to intimidate me."

– Jane Austen

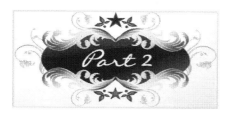

The Serious Stuff

"Courage is resistance to fear, mastery of fear, not absence of fear"

- Mark Twain

There might be a time when using common sense, awareness, diligence, and alertness will not stop the monster. There is a threat percentage that has to be addressed. I want you to be keenly aware and prepared for the chaos that will ensue if that time comes. You need to be in the mindset of understanding that injury will occur. In most of the major crimes that happen there is a high probability of injury. Expect it. Prepare for it mentally, so if and when it occurs it doesn't distract you from your primary goal of getting away. You can save yourself. You just have to believe and act at the first sign of danger.

One of the main things you need to understand is that no two monsters are alike. There are similarities in their behaviors, but their motivations are different. The monster wants you to pay for his bad childhood, that girl in school who jilted him, his twisted views of reality, or something so deep and disturbing he cannot put it into words. The one common thread with all these monsters is that they are looking for weakness. He or she is looking for the girl in white alert mode. The weak girl in this level of attentiveness, who is totally oblivious to what is happening around her, is the one he can surprise and overpower. You, girl, are Fabulous. You already see him coming.

There is also the threat of the familiar beast. You know him and he knows you. He could be an ex, a friend, a neighbor, or a relative. Chances are you have seen this coming. You either chose to ignore the obvious signs or didn't take him seriously. This is your most dangerous situation. This person wants to do YOU harm, not a randomly chosen victim. He has set his sights squarely on you. In the random attacker situation, the one most significant advantage to you is that he couldn't care less if he gets you or the girl next to you. Your familiar attacker wants YOU. You are in his crosshairs. He is thinking about you. He knows your patterns. He is planning. He knows where you live, work, and play. So unless you plan on moving away, the probability of a confrontation is very high. This glitch in your Fabulous life needs to be resolved in order for you to be safe.

The plus here is that you know him, too. You know his name, his face, and his personal information. You probably have a picture you could share with authorities. You are aware of his intentions. Remember, they always leave clues. They are careless that way. It is their downfall. He has already verbalized his anger towards you. He has made threats. He has shown his cards. Notify authorities, family, and friends of the situation you are in. Do not minimize his threats as just hurt and anger. It could be just that, but you aren't going to risk being hurt, so write everything down – the date, a summary of the incident, and who else was around when it happened. It is always better to be safe than sorry.

The unknown attacker vs. the familiar attacker:

- The unknown attacker could choose you at random based on his urge at the moment or he could have noticed you previously and stalked you before making his move.

- The familiar attacker has chosen you as the object of his rage. His sights are set squarely on you.

- The unknown attacker could have a definite plan of attack but usually acts on impulse. It is hard, as a rational thinking person, to understand how someone can act heinously on impulse, but these people aren't wired like you and I. They walk around with ill intent.

- The familiar attacker will usually have a plan or forethought of hurting you specifically. If he snaps, seemingly at random, it is because he has been harboring feelings of anger and rage towards you, so he could have a calculated plan to hurt you or could suddenly hurt you because his rage against you has reached a breaking point.

✓ Defense against a random attacker can range from verbal resistance to extreme physical force to free yourself from the danger of the attack.

✓ Defense against a familiar attacker will usually require an elevated use of force to escape the attack. He will be more aggressive because he knows you and you know him. You can identify him so the risk for him is high. This means he is completely comfortable with his decision to show aggression towards you, regardless of the consequences.

There are no hard and fast rules to define the danger coming, due to the random nature behind the motivation of each monster. The above theories are just that, theories based on the actual crimes of the many convicted criminals I interviewed over several years. Human nature comes into play in real life and the difference between one person and another convicted of very similar crimes could be dramatically different. This section is designed to open your eyes to the potential realities you could face. The monster will not take it easy on you, and you need to have your plan of action ready. You are going to develop the awareness, confidence, and bravery you need with practice. This book is the beginning of your personal journey to enlightenment.

Stalking is defined as the unwanted, obsessive and repeated following and harassing by an individual towards another person.

Stalker!

Stalking

"Evil is powerless if the good are unafraid"
-Ronald Reagan

He is there, watching you, waiting for you, stalking you. He is that ex-boyfriend who can't let go, your ex-husband who made you miserable, the creepy neighbor from down the block, the weird kid from class you helped out with homework because you felt sorry for him, the customer who comes in everyday to sit and watch you work...etc... It is such an eerie feeling to know someone is following your every move. Someone you no longer want to be with, were just friendly with or didn't really know at all, is obsessed with you and won't let you go.

Stalking is defined as the unwanted, obsessive and repeated following and harassing by an individual towards another person. The US Justice Department's Bureau of Justice Statistics reported that 3.4 million persons said they were victims of stalking during a twelve-month period in 2005 – 2006. Women experience twenty stalking victimizations per 1,000 females ages eighteen and older. Victims report approximately 75% of them knew their stalker, 33% say they were followed or spied on, and 21% report being attacked. In a twelve-month period, women are three times more likely to be stalked than raped. Scary statistics.

More recently, the results from the 2010 National Intimate Partner and Sexual Violence Survey conducted by the CDCP found – one in six women in the U.S. have experienced stalking victimization at some point in their lifetime, in which they felt very fearful and believed that they or someone close to them would be harmed or killed.

Identifying a stalker

We come to believe in our mind that a monster looks and acts like a monster and is thus easy to identify. It is simply not true. The Stalking Victimization Report found that 30.3% of stalking is committed by a current intimate such as spouse, boyfriend or former intimate such as an ex-spouse or ex-boyfriend; 45.1% is committed by a known acquaintance such as a friend, roommate, neighbor, classmate, coworker, or relative; 9.7% was committed by a stranger, and in 15% the relationship was unknown.

There are several methods of stalking. Your stalker could:

- ✓ Follow you.

- ✓ Repeatedly call you.

- Spy on you.

- Send you messages or emails.

- Text you.

- Leave you notes.

- Send you unwanted gifts.

- Show up unannounced and without a good reason.

- Wait for you at places such as your work or outside your home or school.

- Spread rumors about you by word of mouth, internet posts or posted in a public place.

- Post compromising or embarrassing pictures of you.

- Harass your family members or friends in an effort to get information about you.

- Kidnap or harm your beloved pet to hurt you.

There are a few ways to keep safe. Follow these safety tips if you feel like you are being stalked:

- Stop all communication and contact with your stalker. In his mind you are in a relationship with him. Responding to a stalker may encourage these thoughts and reinforce their behavior.

- Notify police.

- Always keep your cell phone handy.

- Keep a log of all the incidents, emails, texts, and

save any gifts sent to you. The info will be handy to give to the police and for the courts to give you an order of protection.

✓ Do not go out alone if you can help it.

✓ Change your routines – Take different routes to work, school, the grocery store, the gym or other places you regularly visit.

✓ Trust your intuition.

✓ Have a safe place to go if you feel you are being followed such as a police or fire station, a family or friend's house your stalker doesn't know, a shelter or a public place.

✓ If you are actively being followed, do not go to your home.

✓ Be careful what you post online and make sure to select the highest privacy settings on a public site or forum. Avoid giving personal details about your whereabouts online.

✓ Consider using a nickname instead of your real name to post online.

✓ Carry a weapon of some sort such as pepper spray, mace, a kubotan, a knife etc.

✓ Alert your family, friends, employer, coworkers, school officials, and neighbors about your situation so they can be observant and prepared to assist you.

✓ Give your family, friends, neighbors, coworkers,

and school officials as much information about your stalker as possible – name, pictures, car he drives, where he lives (if known), works, attends school, etc.

◢ Practice vehicle safety – Before you get in your car, look at the back seats and the floorboard behind your front seats. Lock your doors once you get in the car.

◢ Place a credit freeze and fraud alert on your account with the credit bureaus Transunion - 800-680-7289, Experian - 888-690-8086, and Equifax – 800-525-6285.

◢ Identify escape routes out of your home.

◢ Have a stalker bag prepared with your incident log, camera, backup CD with all the info collected and keep it in a safe place so you could grab it when you need it.

◢ Consider having a coworker walk you to your car or a security guard at school walk you to your bus or car.

◢ If all else fails, you might need to consider the drastic move of relocating to stay safe.

High-Tech Stalking

In today's modern age of technology, stalking has evolved into a high-tech new realm and stalkers have found ways to maximize it.

Methods of high-tech stalking

◢ Keystroke logger program installed on your

computer will record your key strokes and store the information in the system or transmit it via the internet.

- ✔ Remotely access your computer or use your email to send messages to others on your behalf.

- ✔ GPS and phone tracking apps can remotely monitor all cell phone activity as well as track your exact location within a few hundred feet.

- ✔ Some software can remotely access a cell phone for information, activate the microphone, listen live to the phone surroundings, and access all text messages.

- ✔ Install wireless video cameras for surveillance.

The technology available to stalk someone is pretty scary, so being aware and knowledgeable is important to being safe. Based on the earlier statistics, we know that most stalkers are close to us and could potentially have easy access to our home. They could also have contact with our electronic devices. Keylogger and remote access programs are virtually undetectable and you will need to install programs to help locate them.

Cell phone spy apps do not have an icon in your screen to locate them. The program is sometimes hidden in the system applications manager so it doesn't seem suspicious. You may notice the phone light up by itself, have trouble turning off, the battery life draining very quickly, or hot to the touch when not in use, this may indicate hidden processes working in the background. Another overlooked indicator is the data usage spike. Compare your monthly data usage to check for changes. High data could indicate your phone is transmitting data such as texts, picture, videos, or emails to another source.

Lastly, it's tough to uncover you're being watched by video surveillance, so you should be aware of any new items in your home or repairs to walls or ceilings. Sometimes your creepy stalker may give it away by saying something that only would be known if he was watching you. Pay attention to the details; monsters will almost always leave clues.

If you feel you have been compromised, let's identify some ways to keep you safe and bring you some peace of mind.

Combating high-tech stalking:

- Install anti-virus and anti-spying software on your computer and keep them updated as malicious software and spyware programs are always changing.

- Password protect your electronic devices and routinely change passwords.

- Back up the data on your phone and perform a factory reset to erase all added programs from your phone. If you are unsure how to do it, contact your service provider tech support for assistance.

- Buy a bug detector. Bug detectors are found at spy shops and are relatively inexpensive. They work by detecting short frequency waves or "electrical noises" emitted by the video device.

✔ Conduct a sweep of your home or surroundings if you feel something is not right. Look for patched walls or freshly painted areas. Notice any new items in your home, such as a stuffed animal, clocks, picture frames, lamps, plants, even pens, etc.

Keep a few things in mind about stalking. There are a number of reasons surveys and studies have found regarding why men stalk women. Here are a few to try to explain, or perhaps for you to identify a reason it may be happening to you. Keep in mind that it is not for you to try to go back and correct. Use it just as a reference.

✔ Retaliation/anger/spite

✔ Control

✔ Mentally ill or unstable

✔ Liked me/found me attractive/had a crush

✔ Keep in relationship

✔ Substance abuser

✔ Stalker liked attention

✔ Proximity/convenience/I was alone

✔ Catch me doing something

✔ Different cultural beliefs/background

✔ Thought I liked the attention

- ✔ Other reasons
- ✔ Don't know why

The long-term effect of stalking is emotional and psychological harm. He is trying to take away your confidence, freedom, and feelings of safety because he wants to control or hurt you. You are magnificent and try as he might, you will identify and deal with him quickly. Notify the authorities, deal with the issue, and protect yourself so you can get on with your fabulous life. You have the strength and the courage to take the necessary steps to get your life back.

Robbery is defined as the felonious taking of the property of another from his or her person or in his or her immediate presence, against his or her will, by violence or intimidation.

Don't take my Coach™!

Robbery

Getting robbed is possibly one of the scariest events anyone could go through. When you are approached by a robber who is demanding your personal items, your instant reaction is to not want to give in. This is a mistake. When approached by someone who is brandishing a weapon, demanding your purse, wallet, laptop, etc., give it to him. You could lose all those items and still walk away with the most valuable property of all: your life. Everything else can be replaced.

Robbery is defined as the felonious taking of the property of another from his or her person or in his or her immediate presence, against his or her will, by violence or intimidation.

There are several types of robberies, so let's review a few:

- Armed robbery – robbery with use of a weapon.
- Strong armed robbery – Using physical force or coercion mostly by multiple assailants.

↙ Pick Pocketing – robbing the victim of money or other valuables from their person without the victim noticing.

The best defense for a robbery is avoidance. Keep your valuables concealed. Staying alert and aware of your surroundings is probably the most tactical way to out-smart a potential robber.

Practice these safety tips when out and about:

↙ Don't walk alone at night if possible. Try to stay in a group or perhaps follow close to a group. There is safety in numbers. Walking alone at night is dangerous for so many reasons. Criminals use the cover of darkness to commit a vast majority of crimes. To a criminal there is a higher likelihood of escape at night. Sometimes we may not have a choice whether to walk at night or not. I don't want you to live in a para-noid, fearful existence, so let's discuss how to be safe and better your odds of not being victim-ized.

↙ Let your best friend or family member know where you are going and the approximate time when you should be home. In today's age of information overload, one bit of information you should be sharing, at least with your friends or family, is where you are going if you are going out alone or with a stranger. I know I said this earlier, but I can't stress enough how time is not on your side if something goes wrong and you need help. If you happen to fall victim and are incapacitated during a robbery, time is of the es-sence in receiving the help you need. Someone needs to know to dispatch help to you within a reasonable amount of time. If no one knows when to expect you back, then you might be waiting for help that isn't coming.

⚐ Walk along well-lit areas – If possible, avoid

"Keep your head up and walk like you're on the red carpet"

*Sgt. Alfredo Dean
Aurora Police Dept.*

wooded areas, heavy bushes, alleyways, vacant lots or other isolated areas. Most horror flicks have at least one scene where an unsuspecting character starts walking alone in an empty alleyway or vacant lot. Ominous music starts to play and inevitably something bad happens. Whenever you are in this situation, where you have a choice whether to take the shortcut through the alley, let the ominous music play in your head to warn you to go the long but safer way.

⚐ When walking on the street, always face traffic. A car could be following you to rob you or kidnap you. If you are walking against traffic, it is more difficult for someone in a car to surprise you. If you have to run, you could run straight, and if they want to pursue you, they will have to turn the vehicle around, giving you time to escape.

⚐ Don't diminish your sense of hearing and awareness with loud music playing in your headphones, texting, or surfing the net while walking. We have all done it — walking or jogging with our headphones on and blasting our favorite music while we ignore everything around us. This is the best way to find yourself on the losing end of a robbery. You are in white alert mode and completely unaware of any potential threats in your surroundings. Don't make yourself an easy target. Keep your music low enough so that you can still hear the ambient noise around you. Keep your eyes open and routinely scanning your surroundings. Also, leave your email alone. If you have something really important that you feel has to be addressed, then stop at a safe, well-lit location and do what you need to do.

- Wear comfortable shoes. When you are out and about, do what all the Fabulous ladies in the city do. Dress to impress and wear comfortable stylish shoes. Everybody in the know knows that trying to walk around in uncomfortable shoes is just ridiculous. Let's be serious, the only reason those models on the cat walk look so effortless as they glide down the catwalk in stilettos, is because they are only walking a short distance on a glass-smooth surface. Stilettos are great, don't get me wrong. I own about 10 pairs but wear them only to dinner parties or other fancy events where I will be sitting most of the time. In everyday life, comfortable shoes that allow you to run if necessary are the real Fabulous girl's friend.

- Keep at least one hand free. Never, ever, walk around with both arms full. Always keep one hand free. Your free hand allows you to access your keys easier, open doors quicker, and give up your purse if you have to quickly. Your main purpose is to get as much distance as possible between you and a robber so the faster you could give him your purse, bag, keys, or whatever your armed monster wants, the quicker he will most likely leave.

"Criminals prey on people that look "scared", normally the ones that walk around with their heads down and don't make any eye contact with anyone. If you look like you belong and aren't afraid to look at them in the eyes the confidence just radiates out of you. The criminals would then fear that you would act on their attack instead of sitting there hopelessly and give them what they want."

Sgt. Alfredo Dean
Aurora Police Dept.

Walk confidently, with purpose, at a steady pace. Look like you know where you are going. Looking confident and aware makes all the difference when you are out in public in so many ways. A confident woman looks prepared and unafraid. The common criminal is looking for a meek, mousy victim. The ones who appear to be easily overwhelmed and controlled. Someone who doesn't look like they would

give much resistance in a robbery. You are secure and powerful looking. He has no idea what you could be capable of, and he is probably not going to try to find out. There are much easier fish to fry and that's the way you like it.

↲ Don't stop to talk to strangers, especially at night. Occasionally a monster will try to break your confident stride by slowing you down with the excuse of asking you a question. Although it may seem rude, give him a polite, "sorry I can't stop" or "I'm in a hurry" and keep moving. You could pretend not to hear him and keep moving. Closely monitor his actions and know if you must pop into the nearest store for safety.

↲ Do not walk into a group of men loitering on the street. If you see a group of guys just hanging out on the street, go the other way. Groups can generate a sense of emotional excitement, which can lead to the provocation of behaviors that a person would not typically engage in if alone. Think about the last sporting event or concert you attended. It's unlikely that you would have been yelling or singing the way you were if you were the only person doing it! The group seems to make some behaviors acceptable that would not be acceptable otherwise. Now look at the bigger picture – a group of guys, testosterone, and the potential for mob mentality to kick in, all provides a recipe for disaster. Cross the street or go another way and just avoid the situation altogether. They are bound to notice your Fabulous nature, so don't invite a possible problem.

↲ Never accept a ride from a stranger or hitchhike. Seriously, this goes without saying. This isn't the '60s and hitchhiking is just an invitation for disaster. If you need a ride, use your cell phone. We are in the age of technology and a friend, relative, or a cab is right at your fingertips. If you get in the car with a stranger, being robbed might be the least of your problems!

ATM safety:

- ⟋ Be aware of your surroundings. If there is someone suspicious looking getting close to you, then cancel your transaction and leave the area.

- ⟋ Avoid using the ATM at night. If you have no other choice, then use it in a well-lit and preferably populated area.

- ⟋ Put your cash away before you step away from the machine. Do not count your cash as you are walking away. That's just begging for trouble.

- ⟋ If you use the drive thru ATMs, then be aware of the area around your car. Lock your doors. You wouldn't want an uninvited creepy passenger sliding into the seat next to you.

Surprise, intimidation, and fear are the key elements of a robbery. Awareness, preparedness, and avoidance are your best defenses. Don't be afraid or embarrassed to leave an area in which you are not comfortable. Keep your valuables hidden and purse closed, especially when you are in an unfamiliar area. Keep a sharp eye out for anything that doesn't seem right to you. Be ready to run. If cornered or surprised, give up your possessions. You will walk away with the most priceless possession of all, your Fabulous life. Everything else can be replaced.

Carjacking is a crime that has become more prevalent. It can also serve as a gateway to more serious crimes such as kidnapping, rape and murder.

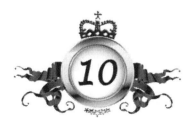

Cars

Carjacking

A crime of opportunity, carjacking has become one of the most rampant crimes in most parts of the world. Carjacking often happens for the sole purpose of taking the car, but there is also a percentage of risk that the act is an opening to a more violent crime. Though carjacking mainly happens at night, if the opportunity presents itself, a criminal will pounce in the daytime, too. Some simple precautions will greatly reduce your chance of falling prey to a creep.

To get a better understanding, there are several reasons carjacking occurs:

- For the sole purpose of stealing the car

- To rob you of your valuables

- To commit a more serious crime such as kidnapping, rape, or murder

- To flee from police

- As a gang initiation

- For some creep's idea of fun

- To strip your car of parts to sell

- To ship your car overseas for profit

Prime target areas for carjackers are intersections, parking garages, shopping malls, grocery stores, gas stations, car washes, ATM machines, residential driveways, special events, concerts, games, parks, highway exit and entry ramps. Basically, anywhere you drive a car is a potential target area. However, the most opportune time to fall victim is when entering or exiting your vehicle.

A few recommended steps to safety:

- Keep a safe distance between you and the car in front of you.

- When stopped at a light or intersection, the tires of the car in front of you should be visible.

- Use either the left turning lane or the middle lane when stopped.

- Keep your doors locked and windows up at stops.

- Avoid isolated roads and parking spots.

- If a minor accident occurs, pull over to a well-lit and busy area.

Bump N Rob

A method used by carjackers is called a Bump n

Rob. In such a scenario, a car will rear-end your vehicle (the "bump"). Usually it is minor but enough to cause you to instinctively jump out of the car to see the damage. The other car will most likely have a passenger who will get out of the car with the driver to see the damage. Once you and the driver are distracted discussing the accident, the passenger will jump in your car and drive off.

Ways to avoid the Bump n Rob:

✔ Before you get out of your car, look around. If something seems suspicious, call the police and wait for them to arrive before exiting your car. Let them know you are in fear, so their response will be quicker.

✔ Remove your keys from the ignition, and grab your purse and your self-defense weapon (pepper spray, kubotan, knife, gun, etc.) before you get out of the car. Your safety defense items will do you no good in the car if you leave them behind.

✔ Quickly make a note of all-important information such as the tag number, vehicle description, and suspect description. Chances are the vehicle they are using is probably stolen, too, so focus on the driver and passenger (if any). Actually, a good idea would be to video tape the confrontation. If you could be discreet, it would be better, but it is a perfect way to document what happened.

✔ Stay alert!

Before getting to your car, you should:

- Have your keys in your hand and ready to unlock your door to get in.

- Walk with purpose and pay close attention to the area around your car.

- If you notice someone hanging around by your car, just keep walking until he is gone. If he is breaking into your car, don't confront him, and call the police.

- Use your phone to record him from a distance.

- Be careful of people who approach you in parking lots to ask for directions, money, or give you flyers.

Once in your car:

- Quickly glance inside before actually sitting down.

- Look at the back seat and the floor behind the front seats.

- Lock your doors. Out of habit we will double click our key remote and inadvertently unlock all the doors in the car. Remember to lock the doors when you get in the car so you don't have any unwelcome guests pop in after you. The best advice would be to try to just click it once so only your door unlocks.

- Pull out of the parking space immediately. Don't linger in your car. It will only attract attention from the wrong person. Chances are, if you are sitting in your car and not moving, it's because you are distracted. Distracted people are easy to surprise and overwhelm.

- Drive on well-travelled and well-lit roads when you can. It may not always be an option, but it is safer to do so when the option is available.

- Leave a safety space between you and the car ahead of you. This way, in case you have to move in a hurry, you don't have to wait for the car to move in order to get away. You could safely zip around the other car. A good distance gauge is when you can see the rear tires of the car ahead of you.

- Check your mirrors often.

- Stay away from the far right lane at night unless you are making a turn. This maneuver makes it more difficult for a potential carjacker to approach your car unnoticed.

- In an extreme situation, you might need to drive through a red light to thwart a carjacker. If you do, be mindful of cars approaching the intersection, so you do not cause an accident.

- Keep your car serviced and in good operating order to avoid breakdowns.

- When you arrive at your destination, keep an eye out for suspicious persons. If you notice someone who looks suspicious, keep driving. Find another spot or come back later.

◢ If you feel threatened, use your horn to attract attention.

Getting out of your car:

◢ Park in a well-lit area and closest to the destination. If you can valet park it will be more favorable. Make sure you are not parked by a dumpster or by any other large object that will obstruct your view. Avoid isolated spots.

◢ Glance around at your surroundings, then get out of the car right away. Sitting in your car will allow a potential threat to sneak up on you.

◢ Do not leave any valuables in view. Move your goodies out of sight, even if your doors are locked. Let's not encourage a jealous creep to break into your car.

Let's imagine you have followed all the safety tips and yet a creep decides to still attack you. Don't resist if he is armed. Give up your car. It is only a possession that can be replaced. Your life is more valuable than a car.

Get away from the car immediately and run! Sometimes, carjacking is a gateway to a more serious crime like kidnapping, rape, or murder, so do everything possible to get away. Do not EVER go with your attacker!

Once you have gotten away, immediately go for help. Make a mental note of what your attacker looks like, as well as any distinguishing marks such as tattoos or birth marks.

Being mentally prepared for a potential attack increases your chances of having a favorable outcome in most cases, no matter what beast you face. Trust your intuition and if something doesn't feel right, get away. Awareness and confidence is key to maintaining a wonderful life.

Kidnapping is a first-step crime. A kidnapper is looking to take you to a secondary spot so he could do a number of things to you. None of these things involve ANYTHING pleasant.

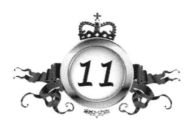

I won't go, You can't make me!

Kidnapping

Imagine this scenario – You are in a dark parking lot, a car drives slowly by, then comes to a stop and a stranger steps out. He asks you a question to make you feel at ease, then he grabs you. What do you do?

You need to fight! You need to scream, scratch, kick, hold on to a stationary item, or claw him in the eyes to get away. Run! Every time your feet hit the ground, you run screaming! He is hoping you are easily overcome so the louder and wilder you are, the better the chances he will back away. Screaming fire has shown to be an effective way to attract attention. Use whatever is at your disposal to hurt him if he is determined and has a tight grip on you. Do whatever you need to do to distract him for a precious chance to get away. We will address different methods of how to defend yourself later in the book.

Statistically, if you are taken, you will not be recovered alive. More specifically, if you make it to the second location, your chances of survival are dismal. I am being brutally honest to make you aware of the gravity of this situation. The truth is that he could do a number of things to get you. He could tell you he promises nothing will happen to you and you will be let go. He is a liar. If he is so bold and desperate to actually lay his hands on you or use a weapon to get you to go with him, he cannot be trusted to keep his promise to let you go. How about you make the decision for him by screaming, causing a scene, and getting away?

He could brandish a weapon and threaten you to make you do as he demands. My suggestion is to always resist. It is highly unlikely he wants to discharge his weapon and attract attention to himself. If he has a knife, you could risk getting stabbed once or twice on the spot and getting away or that same knife could be used to do heinous things to you at the location he is taking you to. By refusing to go you could risk him hurting you there on the spot, but you may get away with your life. If you go with him or get in his vehicle, the chances are almost certain you will not be seen alive again.

There are so many stories of women who have been unprepared when caught in this situation. Although no two cases are exactly alike, one thing is certain — if you don't take decisive action to save your life, you don't have a chance. You need to be brave.

Let's examine the story of Samantha Koenig, an 18-year-old beautiful girl with her whole life ahead of her. She worked at a coffee shack in a parking lot near a busy intersection in her town. One evening at 8 p.m. a man in a hoodie approached the shack and forced her at gunpoint to walk away with him. The whole event was caught on surveillance tape. She walked away calmly with him through a parking lot by a busy intersection and disappeared. After a long exhaustive search by police, family, friends, and volunteers, her body was recovered in a lake by a police dive team a couple months later.

She was clearly unprepared for this surprise attack. What should she have done? Hindsight is 20/20, like the saying goes. If you are aware that things like this could potentially happen to you and you prepare a plan of action, your chances for survival go up substantially. Make up a scenario in your head during your everyday activities, identify the ways you could protect yourself, and get away.

In Samantha's case, she could have possibly run off towards the street screaming when they were in the parking lot. If he had a hold of her, she could have perhaps grabbed hold of the gun and wrestled with him while screaming. You have a better chance if you get into a fight at the initial location than if you are at his chosen (usually secluded) destination. Keep in mind, predators are looking for easy prey. Make yourself a wild cat and become more than he bargained for or can handle. In most cases of random/opportunistic kidnappings, if you are more than what the kidnapper expected, he will possibly retreat. Don't ever give up on yourself. Your life is precious.

My experience working with criminals tells me that working at a coffee shack in a parking lot is not a job for any woman. As a Fabulous girl who is becoming aware of danger and staying away from it, you have to evaluate the whole situation and determine if it is safe for you. This situation is not safe, period. The world we live in is wonderful, but there is a subset of degenerate monsters who share our space. I have met them. They have sick minds and thoughts. They think of bad things to do and evil ways to fulfill their twisted fantasies. This book is a guide to see things from a different perspective, to retrain yourself, to identify danger, and to avoid it.

In the Car

Let's create a different picture. He was able to get you into his vehicle, now what? Try talking to your abductor and gaining trust or sympathy. Use your wit, but no matter what, do not trust him, and if you see an opening to run, take it! This may help and it may give you some insight on his motivation so you could strategize. Be observant of everything around you. You need to get out of there before you get to wherever he is taking you. Let your animal instincts for survival kick in. Do whatever you think will get you free, even if you have to throw yourself out of the vehicle to get away and survive. (Hopefully, if you decide this is the best way at the time to get away, you jump when the car is at a stop, and don't jump in front of an oncoming car.) This is your life. Don't think for a second of giving up on yourself.

If you are placed in the trunk of a car, look at the make, model, color, tag number, and any obvious marks. Be aware, most cars come with a trunk release. Be careful to not pull it too quickly and allow for your attacker to recover you. Perhaps wait until the car is moving or has stopped in traffic or a stop. To clarify: if the car is parked in a parking spot and he has to back out before he can drive away, wait until after he has backed out. You don't want to get run over.

You could also locate the wires to the brake lights

and pull them out or wiggle them if you are unable to find the trunk release. Disabling the lights, or making the lights move, could attract the attention of the police if they happen to pull up behind the car. That is a big IF, so I suggest you try the trunk release.

Strength does not come from physical capacity. It comes from an indomitable will.

Mahatma Gandhi

Try (by all means necessary) not to get tied up. If you can't avoid it, give yourself some wiggle room. A good example is if he is trying to tie your hands behind your back, don't let him pull your wrists together. Leave a gap and tell him you had surgery on your shoulder or elbow and you can't stretch it any closer. This way you could bring your hands to the front. And if there is a gap you could clasp your hands together and possibly remove them from the restraints. If your head is covered, your hands could now be used to remove the blindfold, and perhaps use your teeth to untie yourself if you can't do it otherwise.

If you are in the cab of the vehicle, the situation is better. Jump out screaming at a stop and preferably in a crowded area. Or, at a stop, remove the keys from the ignition and throw them in the back of the car. If you have your seat belt on, yank the steering wheel and cause him to crash into a median, tree, pole, or other inanimate object. If you crash into another vehicle, you risk hurting or killing others. There are plenty of things to hit on the roads that don't involve hurting others.

Start leaving clues behind at every spot you have been – clothing, hair, glasses, blood, spit, or jewelry. Leaving clues will allow rescuers to track you. Rescue dogs have an ability to pick up even the faintest of odors on items and follow the direction in which it leads. The more clues you leave, the easier for them to find you.

Your cell phone could also save your life. Most phones are equipped with GPS and could track you even if they are turned off. Try to always carry your cell on your person so if your purse is dropped or taken away, you still have a way to get help. I suggest you silence your keyboard clicks on your phone so that in case you are in the cab of the car, you could dial or text for help without him hearing the noise. If you can text for help, start by giving information about the vehicle, direction of travel, and attacker before you type "Help! I'm being kid-napped!" This way, if you are discovered and the phone is taken away, there is some crucial info for the police to get started working on. "Help! I'm being kidn" gets them nowhere. Blue Ford Explorer, tag ABC123, gives them a reference point at which to start looking.

If you are in the trunk and you dial for help, remem-ber to keep your voice to a whisper. The aluminum can you are in carries sound and you will be caught. Call the police and start with the description of the car, tag, name, and location where you were taken at first. Then, tell them you are in the trunk. The line is recorded, so getting them the most important information first is vital. If something happens to the communication, the best, most critical information is delivered.

If you were unsuccessful getting way and the attacker has gotten you to the second location, try to keep the phone hidden nearby in case you are searched. When alone, call the police. Snap pictures of the outside of the home from the window, of cars parked out front, of the neighborhood, and send them to family or friends.

Being defeated is often a temporary condition. Giving up is what makes it permanent.

Marilyn Vos Savant

Turn the lights of the room you are in on and off at night repeatedly. Monitor the window to see if your attacker leaves,

and then try to escape. If you see a phone in the home, dial 911 and walk away from the phone. This may have police dispatched to the location to investigate. Most people no longer have phones in their homes, so your cell phone will need to be carefully hidden and used.

It's Personal

In cases of familiar or personal kidnappings the rules are different. This act was probably thought out and planned with you in mind. The beast has targeted you. It is not random and chances are you knew something bad was coming. You perhaps didn't know exactly what, but you were aware of his anger and his threats you chose to ignore.

The most important thing you can do for yourself is to document and report problems with someone familiar such as an ex, a creepy neighbor, a friend, or a family member. Write down every incident and tell a family member or friend. Tell the authorities. Keep your journal in a safe place, or give a copy to someone. Don't dismiss the details. Write down all the places he enjoys, if he or his family has a retreat or cabin somewhere remote, where he likes to go hunting or fishing, and where he likes to go when he just wants to get away. These are the kinds of details that could get the police to you quickly, which could save your life.

Have a safety word or phrase that will alert a relative or friend you are in imminent danger. Let's say if he is in your presence and he allows you to pick up the phone if it rings (because you've convinced him that if you don't pick up they will suspect something is wrong), you casually say the word or phrase and your friend knows to send the police.

Your advantage with this person is that you probably know intimate details about him and certain relationships in his life that you could possibly use to make him think about what he is doing. What is his relationship with his mother? Father? Child? You could possibly work some point about how he would devastate that person if he went to jail or were dead. Be sharp. It's a psychological game. It could possibly buy you time to try to figure out the best way to escape the situation.

Once you have exhausted all measures of trying to get in his head to reason with him and you realize that he is going to try to take you anyway, take off the gloves and use everything you have learned to get away. Save your life. This guy is probably your most dangerous attacker because he knows you know him and there will be no going back once he has crossed the line. He doesn't care. You are not some random person who might not be able to identify him later — you know him. There are no rules here except to say you must do EVERYTHING in your power to protect yourself.

The Parting Gift

If your bad situation gets worst; if you have exhausted all means of escape and are still in his grip; if you have tried your best to outwit him with your smarts or befriend him, gain his sympathy, or pity, and nothing has worked; if you feel that it is possibly the end, then you should scratch and claw your attacker's eyes and skin to get his DNA. Wipe it on your clothing or flick it against walls. Leave your blood and hair everywhere. Fight with every ounce of energy you have and muster up a wild woman. If he is going to end your life, make sure he doesn't get an easy ride. Your clues could get you and your family payback by getting him caught and convicted. Don't let this sick beast get away with what he has done to you. That will be your parting send-off to him.

Kidnapping is a first-step crime. A kidnapper is looking to take you to a secondary spot so he could do a number of things to you. None of these things involve ANYTHING pleasant. He is going to rape you, possibly torture you (sometimes for days), and probably kill you. You cannot give up on yourself. Your life is worth fighting for. I believe in you. You are Fabulous! No monster will EVER take that away no matter what happens.

Fight your intruder at the door or window as he is trying to enter. If he makes it inside your home, you need to carefully evaluate the situation. Keep a cool head, no matter how difficult and scary it is.

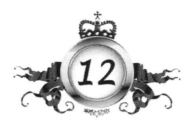

12

This is MY home, not yours!

Home Invasion

Our home is our sanctuary and our safety zone, where we feel like nothing will go wrong. There is a potential for danger lurking everywhere, and you need to be prepared to battle it out. In your sanctuary, have weapons located everywhere so, in a crucial moment, you can reach for something that could save you. It could be that solid bronze figurine on the nook by the door or a decorative rod on the wall.

"Women are like teabags. We don't know our true strength until we are in hot water!"

Eleanor Roosevelt

You know your home and where everything is. You have seen this coming for a long time and have planned for it. You are in control. He is unprepared to deal with you. In his arrogance, he doesn't realize you are smart, prepared, and ready.

Let's imagine a scenario. You are home alone one evening and there is a knock on the door. You look through the peephole and there stands a guy holding flowers. You excitedly open the door. He pushes his way into your home. Now what? We tend to keep the unpleasantries out of our mind. You need to plan. Look around your home right now and think about this scenario. How would you react?

Let's examine what happened to my girlfriend Betty. One night, Betty was at her friend Ty's house enjoying a movie when they heard a knock on the door. Ty went to the door to see who was there. He opened the door and two men burst through. They grabbed Ty and demanded money. Betty was in the living room, which is located at the back of the house. She heard the commotion and carefully looked to see what was happening. She saw two men with guns yelling at Ty. She quietly grabbed her purse and slipped out the back door. Grabbing her purse was a smart move on her part. By doing this she made it seem like there was no one else in the house. Once she was outside, she ran to the neighbor's house and they called the police. The robbers realized there was someone else in the home who had escaped and ran. Outside the home they confronted an armed neighbor who came to the rescue of his friend. A gun battle ensued which resulted in the death of one of the robbers and police capture of the other.

Betty is a smart girl. She didn't panic and kept her cool in this volatile situation. She didn't try to intervene, but instead made her way to safety and got help. How do you feel you would react in this same circumstance?

Having a plan of action is key to safety in a home invasion scenario. Let's look at some prevention basics.

- When pulling up to your home, be aware of anyone loitering around. Keep driving if you must, or notify the authorities.

⌁ Fortifying your home is a necessity to being safe.

⌁ Inspect your doors and windows monthly to check for breaks.

⌁ Install a strike plate box to your door to make sure it is secure. Check the locks on your doors and windows to make sure they are operational and secure.

⌁ Install a wide view peephole to get a better look at who is knocking at your door.

"Develop an 'action plan' in the event you are confronted with an emergency. Role play scenarios in your mind"

Rafael Torres
Torres Protection Group

⌁ Never just open the door when someone is knocking.

⌁ Chain locks are ineffective as a way of keeping a safe zone between you and an intruder. Being able to identify the person at the door before you open it is important. Talk through the door, if you must, to the person knocking before you risk opening the door

Alarms

Have an alarm installed with a siren....a very loud siren. Those sirens are effective in disorienting and discouraging most criminals. Have panic buttons installed in a couple places in your home. They could be silent and notify the police or set off the siren while notifying the police. I recommend placing one by the front door and one in your bedroom. Don't forget to have your alarm decal on your front window. Surprisingly, this will act as a deterrent when criminals are selecting a home to target.

Action Plan

Next have a plan of action with your neighbors. Introduce yourself to your neighbors. Be friendly. In a crisis, your neighbor could help save your life. Have a plan of action with your family. Discuss plans with your children. Chances are, if a home invasion is going to take place, your whole family will not be in the same room of the house or apartment. Teach your kids that it is OK to jump out of a window if it's on the first floor. We get so accustomed to looking at windows as barriers when in fact they are just decorative accessories that let light into your home. Unless you have bullet-proof glass for windows, most windows just open so you could get out or break it, if you must, to escape. If your bedrooms are located on the second floor, every room should have a rope ladder. In case of fire or robbery, the family could get out safely.

Perhaps you could train your kids to activate the panic button if they hear a commotion. Discuss different scenarios and make plans. Keep in mind that no two robberies will be exactly the same and even the best thought-out plan can fail. You have to look at the situation, keep a level head, and plan your response as it unfolds.

The Fight

Fight your intruder at the door or window as he is trying to enter. If he makes it inside your home, you need to carefully evaluate the situation. Keep a cool head, no matter how difficult and scary it is. If you are alone, try to gauge what the intent is. Is he after money, is it personal, or is it to possible rape or physically injury you? Always try to escape. Sometimes, if you appear to comply, this may work in your favor. Your intruder may let his guard down and you can escape or strike him. If you decide to strike him, do it quickly and with as much force as you can to stun or incapacitate him; then run!

If there are children in the house, you definitely need to keep your cool. Training your kids to respond quickly by practicing their escape plan is essential to ensuring their safety. Teach them to ignore what the intruder might say to keep them there. He may tell them that if they run he will hurt you or kill you. Make them ignore those threats and activate the panic alarm, or run to safety anyway.

Keep thinking about and evaluating your possible chances as the events unfold to determine what your response will be. Do not allow yourself to be tied up. If that is something your intruder plans on doing, then it is time for you to talk your way out of it or fight. Think about it this way, if he is taking his time to tie you up, then this is going to be a long event. You need him out of there as quickly as possible for the safest outcome. Time is not on your side. If he sets up camp inside your home, your risk of injury goes up.

Be Observant

Based on your particular set of circumstances, perhaps you decide that being compliant is a better choice for your scenario. Be very observant of everything going on. Take note of the robber's race, height, age, approximate weight, scars, tattoos, clothing, hair color, eye color, complexion, and note anything unusual about him or them. If they touch anything bare handed do not touch it and make a mental note of it. When they are done and leave, look at what vehicle they are in. Remember the make, model, color, and any special features. Notice in which direction they travelled. Lock up immediately and call police.

Home invasions are extremely frightening, but if you keep a level head and stay calm, your outcome may be OK.

Rape is an act of anger, violence and control, not of passion. Sex is the weapon used to degrade you and to make him feel powerful.

When NO means NO!

Rape

"Every 2 minutes someone in the U.S. is sexually assaulted"

-R.A.I.N.N. – Rape, Abuse & Incest National Network

As a woman, this is the hardest topic to discuss. It is the type of intimate crime that is meant to degrade you and strip you of your Fabulous confidence. Not you. You know the beast and are ready. Understand that rape can happen at almost any time. I say that because your beast could be a stranger on the street or the man lying next to you in bed. He could be the ex-boyfriend you left, the man you are currently with, a friend, a relative, a neighbor, or almost anyone.

I want you to be as prepared as possible. If it is a familiar rape, chances are you have seen it coming and have just refused to see it for what it actually is. Likely there have been subtle or not-so-subtle hints he has given you. Your alert level is always at orange when he is around. Learning to trust your intuition will help you stay clear of a bad situation. Do not dismiss your feelings; they are your inner guidance system, perfectly tuned to keep your wonderful life on course.

"Every two minutes someone in the U.S. is sexually assaulted." What a startling and sobering statistic. Every two minutes translates to 207,754 victims of sexual assault per year. Eighty percent of those victims will be under the age of 30. Those are the average annual numbers reported by the Rape, Abuse & Incest National Network. In 2010, the Department of Justice reported 268,574 sexual assaults/rapes in the U.S. Of those, 253,555 were against women.

Let's break it down further:

- Intimates (intimate relationships)   109,205
- Relatives   12,921
- Well-Known/Casual Acquaintances   82,102
- Strangers   41,948
- Did not know relationship   3,391

Rape is an act of anger, violence and control, not of passion. Sex is the weapon used to degrade you and to make him feel powerful. The above statistics indicate a sobering reality. Rapists are not just strangers lurking in alleyways; they are potentially lying next to you in bed. The familiar rapist is known to you. He is a boyfriend, husband, ex, relative, friend, or acquaintance. It is a sad reality to face, but the sooner you decide to see the possibilities, the sooner you could protect yourself.

There are many myths to address in regards to rape:

- You invited a rape.
- What you were wearing, and the way you were acting, caused you to be raped.
- Only attractive young women get raped.
- Rapists are weird-looking monsters who act bizarrely.

- Rapists are always strangers.
- Rapes only take place at night.

Here are some true facts about rape:

- You did not invite a rape.
- What you wear and the way you act doesn't cause someone to rape you.
- All women are subject to being raped. Age doesn't matter to a monster.
- Rapists come in all types. They are handsome and gallant as well as ugly and mean.
- Some rapists are strangers, but a huge number are familiar faces – boyfriend, husband, ex, friend, relative, or neighbor.
- Although a good portion of rapes happen at night, an overwhelming number occur in the daytime.
- 50% of rapes happen in the home or general vicinity.
- Most rapists are not armed when they commit a rape.
- Most are planned in advance.
- Most are never reported because the victim feels either too afraid or that she was at fault.
- It is never your fault. Do not allow a rapist monster to convince you that, had it not been for your actions, sexy dancing, drinking, staring, or provocative clothing, you wouldn't have been victimized.

According to esteemed Psychologist Nicholas Groth, author of *Men who Rape: The Psychology of the Offender*, who over a 25-year period observed, studied, and counseled over 3,000 rapists, surmised that rapists fall into three motivation categories:

✔ Anger rape is the unpremeditated attack and, therefore, he may not be fully committed to the attack. He may be deterred by resistance, although resistance may also fuel his anger, as he may feel you are stopping him from getting what he wants.

✔ Power rape is usually committed by men who feel insecure, or have doubts about their competence. This is their way of feeling in control. The power category rapist searches for unsuspecting or timid victims. Victims who fight back better know exactly what they are doing because he is attacking to prove himself a man and his self-esteem is on the line. If you take the chance to fight, you had better make it count.

✔ Sadism rape, also known as sadistic rape, is committed by someone who is excited by acts of forcible sex, and by someone who doesn't achieve the level of satisfaction he desires from consensual sex. The method he uses is torture, and he will use instruments to rape. He is interested in terrorizing and inflicting long-lasting harm. Active resistance from his victim will fuel his enjoyment and may incite him to further acts of depravity to illicit more response.

Rapists are then categorized in four types:

✔ Anger-Retaliatory Rapist – This rapist's characteristics commonly include drug or alcohol abuse, severe anger issues, or impulsive behavior problems. He has a hatred for women and wants to make them pay for some past wrong done to him. His attacks are usually spontaneous and vicious. He probably does not intend to kill his victim, but may beat her to death if she resists. Other characteristics are a below-average I.Q. and he usually leaves behind a sloppy crime scene. He accounts for 28% of rapes.

- Power-Reassurance Rapist – Known as the "gentleman rapist" by law enforcement, he is the least violent of all the attackers. His victims are familiar to him, and may be a friend or neighbor. He often fantasizes about a consensual relationship with the victim, as opposed to the act of rape. He is the "Peeping Tom"-type stalker who watches his victims. He often takes trophies of the attack such as panties or bras. He is of average intelligence, socially inept, and unable to develop romantic relationships. He does not intend to hurt his victim, who he sees as his lover, although the possibility exists that he may turn violent, but will most likely not resort to any serious attack. If he tells you he will return to make sure you are OK, have the police waiting — he is highly likely to return. He accounts for 27% of rapes.

- Power-Assertive Rapist – He is the most common type of rapist. For him, rape is a way to validate his machismo and testosterone. He feels superior to women. He is loud, rowdy, and considers himself a man's man. He works in some kind of male-dominated field. His hunting ground is usually a bar or club where he will employ a variety of cons to get women to leave with him, such as offering to walk her to her car or offering a ride home. His attack is meant to degrade and humiliate his victim and assert his dominance. His attacks will be verbal and physical, although he does not intend to kill his victim. He is arrogant and doesn't hide his identity. He accounts for 40% of rapes

- Anger-Excitation Rapist – He is the most dangerous rapist. He intends to torture his victims and often murders them. He is calculating and will often carry a "rape kit" with tools used to kidnap, torture, and inflict great pain on his victim. He has a meticulously thought-out fantasy in his mind and is very careful to clean up after his attack. He is intelligent and educated, and tries to conceal his identity at all costs. He accounts for 5% of rapes.

Your first defense against a rape is realizing that it can happen to you. Your age, attractiveness, social status, money, or intelligence does not matter. You need to admit to yourself that you are at risk. Have a safety plan. Keep yourself informed, and have a back-up plan for your safety plan.

The reality is that your instincts could help identify your threats, but you have to listen to them. Avoidance is the best defense against a rape. Make your safety your top priority. Let's address some everyday scenarios to examine ways to stay safe.

In your car, remember all the safety tips I previously discussed in the earlier sections and:

- If your car breaks down, call a tow truck and remain in your car with the windows up until help arrives.

- Do not get out of your car if someone pulls over

to help you and, although it may seem rude, talk to them through the window, especially at night. If your phone isn't working, ask them to call a tow truck for you. On a hot day, reject their offer to sit in their cool car.

↙ Don't turn into your driveway if you feel you are being followed. Keep driving past your house and to a well-populated area or a police station.

Since most rapes occur in or around your home, take a good look around your place and follow some good tips:

↙ Check your doors, windows, and locks to determine how durable they are. Add a strike plate box on your door to help prevent break-ins.

↙ Make sure your alarm is in good working order. If you rent and don't have an option for installing an alarm, there are many battery-operated door and window alarms you can buy.

↙ Don't put your name on your mailbox. If you do, only use your last name and include another last name to make it seem as if more people are living there.

↙ Get a wide-angle peep hole to see who is knocking. Don't automatically open a door.

↙ Do not rely on chain locks, they are easily compromised. The solid bolt ones are better. It's better to just talk through the door.

↙ Ask for identification from people coming into your home to do service and have someone else present in the home, too.

Your favorite bar or club is prime hunting grounds for creeps, but following a few savvy tips could keep your good time secure. Several of these are covered in earlier chapters, but they are totally worth repeating:

- Valet park or always park in a well-lit spot closest to the venue.
- Have a Fabulous friend or friends with you.
- Know your limits with alcohol, and never do drugs.
- Keep your drink in your possession at all times. If someone offers to buy you a drink (even if it is soda), have them order it in your presence and take it directly from the waiter or bartender's hands.
- If you start to feel woozy or weird, find a friend immediately. Find a staff member and tell them you think you've been drugged and not to let the guy take you if you pass out.
- Never walk outside a club with a guy to "talk" because it's too loud inside.
- Never accept a ride from someone you just met and don't really know.
- Don't let a pushy, aggressive guy make you do something your instincts are telling you not to do. Your safety is a hundred times more important than his feelings.

When you are dating someone, remember, you decide whether you are ready or not to have sex with him. Do not let a man push you into doing something you are not ready for or comfortable doing. Even if you have already had sex with him, it doesn't mean you can be forced to have sex again or at his whim. Having the title of boyfriend or husband does not mean that person has the right to physically violate you. Forcing sex upon you is rape and should not be tolerated. You are fabulous and have the absolute right to refrain from having sex. No one should make you feel pressured to do something you don't want to do. If your boyfriend cannot respect your boundaries, then show him the door. Next!

Best Defense

This is a tough one. There are so many variables and types of rapists. Experts have disagreed for years as to what the most effective response from a victim should be. If you are unable to avoid the situation altogether, then you have to figure out which category of rapist you have on your hands. You must also determine what the best option is in your circumstance. What are your chances of escape? Is there a weapon involved? Are you somewhere you could possibly attract attention with your screams? Can you outwit him? Do you have the ability to incapacitate him? Are you willing to do what it takes to survive? All these questions can only be answered by you, and only you, when you are in the thick of it.

Ted Bundy, inarguably one of the most prolific rapist-murderers in U.S. history, was a classic example of a sadism/anger-excitation rapist. He was handsome, educated, had a bad childhood, and was meticulous, manipulative, and exceptionally perverse. His victim count was between 30–36+. He used his looks as a way to con girls into trusting him. Most all of his targets were raped and murdered. He used a "rape kit" with various disguises and instruments of torture to inflict pain on his victims. He had every characteristic described by Groth and FBI profilers about the sadistic rapist. These people exist and are counting on your trusting, compassionate nature to harm you.

Education is a powerful weapon that could change your world for the better. Commit yourself to enjoying every minute of the process.

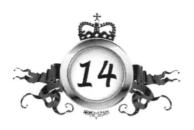

School Daze

Campus Crimes

A study conducted by the National Crime Justice Service, called The National College Women Sexual Victimization study, was commissioned by the U.S. Department of Justice to expand on the limitations of the current limited studies. The study expanded the currently available reports by employing a wider nationally represented sample of college women. They assessed a greater range of sexual crimes to include stalking. The study provides a depth in questioning and research that was not available previously.

The study found that college (or university) campuses host large concentrations of young women who are at greater risk for rape and other forms of sexual assault than women in the general population or in a comparable age group. The researchers found that, at a college that has 10,000 females, students could experience 350+ rapes a year.

Additionally, the study indicated that nine out of ten victims knew their offender:

- 35.5% were committed by classmates
- 34.2% by friends
- 23.7% by a boyfriend or ex-boyfriend
- 2.6% by an acquaintance
- 4% other

The study shows that fewer than 5% of the rapes, or attempted rapes, were reported. There are a number of reasons why. Researchers found the victims:

- Didn't want family or others to know
- Perceived lack of proof the incident happened
- Were not clear it was a crime, or that harm was intended, or that it was serious enough
- Fearful of the police response or lack of response, as well as hostile treatment from the justice system
- Fearful of retaliation by the attacker or others

Thirteen percent of females in the study report they had been stalked since the school year began. Stalking is a huge factor in this study versus the more limited one, because the study gives a broader definition of stalking. Stalking is a first step in a crime being committed. "Although some victims reported being physically injured, the most common consequence was psychological: Almost 3 in 10 women said they were 'injured emotionally or psychologically' from being stalked. In 15.3 percent of incidents, victims reported that the stalker either threatened or attempted to harm them. In 10.3 percent of incidents, the victim reported that the stalker 'forced or attempted sexual contact.'"

The U.S. Congress passed the Student Right-to-Know and Campus Security Act of 1990, also known as the Jeanne Clery Act. This legislation mandates that colleges and universities participating in Federal student aid programs "prepare, publish, and distribute, through appropriate publications or mailings, to all current students and employees, and to any applicant for enrollment or employment upon request, an annual security report" containing campus security policies and campus crime statistics for that institution (see 20 U.S.C. 1092(f)(1)).

The law was amended in 1992 to add a requirement that schools afford the victims of campus sexual assault certain basic rights, and was amended again in 1998 to expand the reporting requirements. The 1998 amendments also formally named the law in memory of Jeanne Clery. Subsequent amendments in 2000 and 2008 added provisions dealing with registered sex offender notification and campus emergency response. The 2008 amendments also added a provision to protect crime victims, "whistleblowers", and others from retaliation.

Jeanne Clery was a 19-year-old university freshman when her parents dropped her off at school after spring break in 1986. Five days later she was murdered by a fellow student in her on-campus dorm room. Jeanne's killer was Joseph Henry, who boasted and bragged about her murder to friends. Jeanne had been beaten, raped, sodomized, strangled, and mutilated with a broken bottle. Although she lived in a secure dorm, which had 3 automatic-lock security doors, students would often prop the doors open with pizza boxes for ease of access. Henry took advantage of this lapse in judgment and safety to gain entry to attack Clery. When police arrested him, he had Jeanne's property in his possession.

Jeanne's parents did not just sit back and silently mourn their daughter. They took a proactive approach and lobbied state lawmakers for statutes requiring colleges and universities to publish campus crime reports. They also started Security on Campus (SecurityonCampus.org) a non-profit, dedicated to preventing violence, substance abuse, and other crimes on college and university campuses across the United States, and to compassionately assist the victims of these crimes.

The Clery Act requires colleges and universities to:

- Publish an Annual Security Report (ASR).

- Have a public crime log.

- Disclose crime statistics for incidents that occur on campus, in unobstructed public areas immediately adjacent to or running through the campus, and at certain non-campus facilities.

- Issue timely warnings about Clery Act crimes, which pose any serious or ongoing threats to students or employees.

- Devise an emergency response, notification, and testing policy.

- Compile and report fire data to the federal government and publish an annual fire safety report.

- Enact policies and procedures to handle reports of missing students.

While rape is certainly something to think about on campus, be aware that a number of other crimes happen on campus, too. A huge problem is burglary. Burglary is the act of breaking into a structure for the purpose of committing a crime. No great force is needed to gain entry (such as pushing open a door or slipping through an open window). The entry of the structure is unauthorized. While the most common reason for a burglary is theft, it can be applied to a variety of crimes in which unauthorized entry was made in order to commit the second criminal act. Other crimes to be aware of on campus are robbery, aggravated assault, and motor vehicle theft.

Now that I have managed to scare you (not my intention; I just want you to know the facts) let's keep you safe!

Personal Safety

- Be aware of your surroundings – Stay in F.A.B. mode at all times. While walking from class to class and building to building keep your senses aware of what is going on around you at all times.

- Keep your keys with you at all times – You need to have the ability to quickly get in to your Residence Hall. If your keys get lost, just pay the fine and get a new set. You can't depend on your roommate to keep letting you in. Your keys may pop up, but then again, they may just be lost and no amount of hoping is going to bring them back. Actually, if you have any identifying information on the keys, you should probably get your locks changed.

- Have a defense item with you at all times (decide which one is best for you, be it pepper spray, a kubotan, or a mini horn), and have it always available to help you in a flash.

- ↲ Don't leave your items alone in the library – even if for a moment while you run to the restroom. If it is important, take it with you. Theft can happen in a second.

- ↲ If you have a car, always keep it locked – Don't make it easy for someone to take your stuff, car, or wait for you to get in to take you.

- ↲ Check on your car weekly if you don't use it often –Just because you don't use it, doesn't mean someone else isn't having fun.

- ↲ Have an electronic lock on your laptop, desktop, and cell phone – Just in case, all your data is secure.

- ↲ Activate your GPS app on your cell phone – This handy app will help locate your phone if it goes missing or is stolen. The real benefit is that if you go missing with your phone, the police will be able to locate you quicker, perhaps saving your life.

- ↲ Put at least three I.C.E. numbers on your phone – I.C.E. means In Case of Emergency. Make one of these three people someone with decision-making abilities over your health, and someone local. Include the letters I.C.E. after their name on your phone so if you are incapacitated, police or medical personnel call them for you.

- ↲ Have a friend with you when going out at night – Being on a campus setting seems so safe and a pseudo-utopia of cool, but always having a friend with you while you are out at night will provide you a safety not achieved while alone.

Predators look for single, vulnerable women. There is strength in numbers and two is usually more than a monster wants to deal with.

◢ When traveling around campus at night, have an escort – If you must get somewhere quick and can't find a friend to go with you, call the campus escort service. It might seem lame, but consider the option of getting hurt instead. How lame is that?

◢ Know where the emergency phones are located on campus – Thankfully there are emergency phones with blue lights shining. When in need, pick up the phone and call!

◢ Always tell a friend where you are going and when you expect to be returning, as well as with who – If something happens to you, the quicker someone can get you help the better. If no one knows you are missing, then you could be in trouble.

◢ Know the number to Campus Safety or the Campus Police Department – Every campus has them so get to know them.

Dorm Safety

◢ Notify someone if the security doors in your residence hall do not work properly – What happened to Jeanne Clery could have possibly been avoided if the Hall doors were locked like they were supposed to be. Keep your new temporary home safe by making sure those locks always work. Notify security if the locks are inoperable or have been tampered with.

⏋ Don't let someone into your residence hall you don't know – You might come off as rude. You might get a nasty stare, but tough. If you don't know them, then don't let them in. If they lived there, they'd have keys. Let them ask security to let them in. You wouldn't let a stranger into your house just because he wanted in, so shut the door behind you and keep walking.

⏋ Keep your dorm room and windows locked at all times – You wouldn't want a monster sneaking in. Even if you are just running out for a quick shower, lock it.

⏋ Install an alarm on your door and window – There are a variety of simple alarms you can attach to your windows and doors that will alert you to someone sneaking in. It will probably even scare them off. Better to be safe than sorry.

⏋ Have a safety plan with your neighbors – Be friendly with those living around you. In an emergency, they could be valuable help.

⏋ If you live off campus, have a check-in friend – Living away from the campus makes it a little more challenging for people to notice you. On campus, everyone is socializing and knows everyone who is always around them, so it is easier to know when someone is missing. Off campus, dwellers should have a friend they are comfortable with to check on each other daily.

Campus Party and Game Safety

⏋ Go with friends – Parties and games are so

much more fun when you've got your friends with you!

✔ Have at least one nondrinking friend – Every group needs that one awesome friend who is sober and is going to keep you out of trouble.

✔ Don't feel pressured to drink – Stay away from alcohol if you are underage. Not a popular statement, but honestly the best advice. Aside from being illegal, colleges and universities have such strict policies on the matter, you could end up getting expelled and lose out on so much. It really isn't worth it. The strongest thing you could do for yourself is to learn to speak up and stand up for yourself and stay out of trouble. There is plenty of time in your life; you will legally be able to do what you want to do. Patience.

"It takes a great deal of bravery to stand up to our enemies, but just as much to stand up to our friends"

JK Rowlings

✔ Serve your own drinks, or if there is a bartender, take the drink directly from him/her even if it's water – The reality is, there are bad people who want to do bad things. Don't give them the chance to slip something into your drink, even water.

- Keep your drink with you at all times (see above).

- Stay away from drugs – Aside from being illegal, they are incredibly harmful to your Fabulous life. You have an amazing future ahead of you. Don't take chances on hurting yourself and your brilliant mind.

- Don't leave the party without your friends – Just as you wouldn't want to be left behind, don't leave anyone else behind. Be a good friend, and help everyone home. Wouldn't you feel terrible if you left someone behind and they got hurt?

- Don't leave the party with a guy you don't know very well or at all – One-night stands are tacky and gross. What is even worse, is getting raped. Stay safe. If someone is interested in you, they will take their time to get to know you and not pressure you into something you are not ready for.

- If you start to feel woozy or sick, get to a friend immediately – Most "date rape" drugs have virtually no color or taste, but they will knock you out quickly, so if you start to feel funny or woozy, get to a safe place or person right away. You will have only minutes before you are rendered unconscious.

- At a game or a party, if the crowd starts to get rough or too rowdy, get away. Drinking + testosterone + adrenaline + crowds of people = potential danger. If you see a group of people getting out of control, move away. Don't pull out your camera to record the mayhem, just move on.

There are psychology theories surrounding mob mentalities and the bottom line is, it is dangerous. One drunk guy decides to turn his attention towards you, and you could find yourself getting sexually assaulted and touched inappropriately. Now you are standing there, embarrassed, wondering what to do. This exact scenario is what then causes women to doubt themselves as to what is a sexual assault, and wonder if she caused it by being there ... a slippery slope. Your personal space should NEVER be invaded by anyone you did not invite in. Being drunk is not an excuse to lay hands on anyone.

- Never get into a car with someone who has been drinking. Take a stand and be safe.

Guide yourself by these simple rules, be confident, be observant, and you should have a great and safe time in college. Everything may not always be perfect, but you have a great start to creating a wonderful life for yourself.

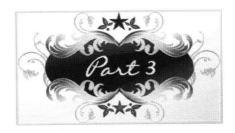

Stilettos are off and it's time to rock!

"If someone tries to kill you, you don't have the option of averting your eyes or changing the subject. You are forced to deal with that person's behavior. The experience is in fact a loss of certain illusions. The world is not how you want it to be, it is the way it is. There are bad people in the world and they need to be stopped."

– Michael Crighton – The State of Fear

"The world is not how you want it to be, it is the way it is," can be a difficult statement to accept. There are bad people in this world. They have bad intentions. Their minds do not process information the same way as you and I. They have no sympathy, no empathy — only rage. They are just bad, and some are evil. A monster will not fight fair – he does not care about your feelings or how much he hurts you. He could do a number of terrible things to you and not even lose sleep about it.

You need to be prepared to discover your inner heroine, who is truly the only one you can turn to in a time of crisis. She is inside of you and she is fierce. She loves you like no one else and wants you to be safe. She only needs one thing from you: permission. Grant yourself permission to act with complete and utter unchained ferocity, to put an end to the threat and escape the situation. Think about this - when a heroine shows up in a movie, does she just survive or does she win? She wins every time, because just surviving means having to deal with the physical and psychological aftermath of an attack. So the heroine uses everything in her power to make sure the threat is dealt with ferociously, allowing her to escape, so she can go back to her perfect life.

Your inner heroine needs tools to do this for you, and it is up to you to explore which ones you feel will work best for you. A time may come where it is only you and a monster. You decide what your reaction will be. No one else can make the choice for you. No one else will live with the consequences but you. Will you decide to unleash your heroine? I believe you have the power. Let's seek out the best method of action for you.

> *"You never know how strong you are until being strong is the only choice you have."*
>
> *Unknown*

-

I learned to control and focus my anger and aggression. I was no longer going to be his victim. The next time I saw my monster, he knew. No words needed to be spoken. Perhaps it was my stoic, yet menacing, glare that let him know his days of being in charge were over.

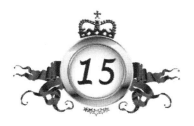

15

Be Powerful

Self-Defense

We all need to discover how to be powerful. Martial Arts is very near and dear to me. It helped me get through some of the hardest times in my life. My girlfriend, Liz, who I refer to as my undercover angel, turned my life around in the most significant way. I was in turmoil in my teen years. The monster I referred to early in the introduction was still in my life, hurting me. He had been doing it in one form or another since I was a little girl. I was at the breaking point, and it was reflected in my everyday life. My relationship with my family and friends was suffering. My school work was suffering. My conduct and behavior was just one cross look away from a violent outburst. At my worst, I once picked up a desk in the middle of class and threw it. I had no confidence and was bubbling up with anger.

I will never forget the day she asked me if I wanted to join her at a karate class. I jumped at the chance. As a little girl, I used to watch old Kung Fu movies and daydream I was the fierce heroine on TV. I remember the first night of class, as I stood in formation with my shorts and tank top, looking at everyone so effortlessly doing these amazing arm and hand movements. Striking and punching. Spinning and kicking. A large bag hung from the ceiling and made a distinct popping noise when struck by a powerful kick. This was right up my alley. I could vent my frustrations in a safe and cathartic way. No longer would I have to punch and scream into my pillow to get my anger out. Little by little, through the teachings and extra effort of my wonderful instructor, my anxieties diminished. My spirit was lifted. But most importantly, my confidence started blossoming. I felt powerful on the inside, in my soul. With everything I learned and every competition that I won, I felt a boost.

I learned to control and focus my anger and aggression. I was no longer going to be his victim. The next time I saw my monster, he knew. No words needed to be spoken. Perhaps it was my stoic, yet menacing, glare that let him know his days of being in charge were over.

This place was where my new chance at life began. I learned so much about myself, gained confidence, and realized for the first time in my life that I was powerful. I discovered my inner strength and heroine. Fabulous, you can, too. Go sign up for a self-defense class. There are so many choices of wonderful disciplines to learn.

Here are some choices for you to pick:

- ⌐ MMA – Mixed Martial Arts - MMA was believed to date back to the ancient Olympic Games in 648 B.C., when pankration — the martial training of Greek armies—was considered the combat sport of ancient Greece. In recent years it resurfaced in Brazil via a combat sport known as vale tudo ("anything goes"). Mixed Martial Arts is, just as the name suggests, a mix of different styles of martial arts, combined to create a hybrid versatile fighting method. In the early 90's, when it first made its appearance in the United States, it was a male only sport. In recent years, women have made a significant impact in the art. We are taking charge and proving ourselves very capable of perfecting the techniques used in this very devastating sport. Women such as Gina Carano and Munah Holland, who have taken the sport to a whole new level and proven that women can do anything.

- Jiu-jitsu – Jiu-jitsu, also known as "gentle, flexible or pliable art", is a method of fighting that makes use of few or no weapons and makes use of holds, throws, and powerful strikes to subdue an attacker. The goal of jiu-jitsu is simple: to disarm or disable an attacker by using their own forcefulness against them. Jiu-jitsu is a style designed for close combat defense to defeat an armed or unarmed attacker. The art evolved among the warrior class (samurai) in Japan, centuries ago. It was a particularly brutal fighting method of the time, designed to cripple or kill an opponent The Jiu-jitsu system of fighting employs the techniques of fist strikes, kicking, kneeing, throwing, choking, immobilizing holds, and use of select weapons. The essential theory of the system is the concept of "gentle or pliable" bending or yielding to an enemy's direction of attack while attempting to control it. Essentially using the attacker's own momentum or motion to guide them in a direction you prefer, to be able to control them. Also employing the use of the hard or tough parts of the body such as knees, fists, elbows, and knuckles against an enemy's vulnerable spots. Other techniques taught include throwing, striking, restraining by pinning and strangling, joint locks, grappling, and weaponry. The art is best known for its effectiveness against weapons, use of throws, and its locks such as leg locks, arm bars, and wrist locks. A relatively newer method of jiu-jitsu is the Brazilian style. If your goal is to be able to defend yourself competently, Brazilian Jiu-jitsu has significant advantages over most other martial arts. It is the one style that covers all areas of fighting completely without the need for cross-training. Brazilian Jiu-jitsu was designed as a fighting style to make up for what was lacking in other styles and make a complete style. Basically, it was designed to defeat other martial arts styles. Several other styles specialize in striking, but none of them have adequate response for someone who is pinned on the ground. Brazilian Jiu-jitsu offers solutions for defending against striking attacks while standing and on the ground, in addition to all methods of grappling attacks. Most

"Mastering others is strength, Mastering yourself is true power."

- Lao Tzu

fights end up on the ground. Being able to properly respond and defend yourself is crucial to you getting free and running away. Imagine the look of surprise on your monster's face if he takes you down and you apply an arm lock or a choke hold on him? He messed with the wrong diva!

- Krav Maga – Krav Maga translates to "Contact Combat or Close Quarter Combat." Krav Maga teaches students to rely on their natural instincts and reflexes for self-defense. Awareness, confidence, and mental conditioning are fundamental to Krav Maga training. Krav Maga's philosophy is, never to do more than necessary, but to react with speed, economy of motion, and the appropriate measure of force. Speed is vital, and students are taught to strike instinctively at the human body's vulnerable parts. The key basic principle is to finish the fight as quickly as possible. It, therefore, focuses emphasis on the most vulnerable parts of the body such as the neck, groin, eyes, face, etc. Krav Maga is dynamic and constantly evolves as situations require. A common lesson learned is to "always use the nearest tool for the job." The system teaches students to maintain awareness of their surroundings while dealing with a threat in order to look for escape routes, identify other attackers, and identify objects that could help defend against the attacker. The system has been tested in battle and on the streets for years. One important lesson in Krav Maga emphasizes that there are no rules on the street. If a situation is dire, the defender must do whatever is necessary to overcome the threat. This may include a finger planted into an eye, shouting into an attacker's ear, or a head butt or a bite to the neck. Krav Maga uses the concept of "retzef," Hebrew for "continuous motion," to complete a defense. Krav Maga uses the same building blocks from the simplest defenses to the most advanced techniques, including empty-handed defenses and disarms against bladed weapons, firearms, and even rocks. Krav Maga is world-renowned for its disarming techniques against assailants posing a threat with weapons. Krav Maga is designed for people of all shapes, sizes, and physical abilities, regardless of age. While Krav Maga was designed to teach soldiers to become proficient in hand-to-hand combat tactics in a short time, the same is true of Krav Maga's civilian adaptation. Krav Maga is well received within law enforcement and military circles. Women have been training for years in Krav Maga. The training is used to empower women to defend themselves no matter what danger they may face.

- Boxing - boxing contestants try to land blows hard and often with their fists, each attempting to avoid the strikes of the opponent. While not historically a women's sport, more and more women have made their mark and slowly integrated into the sport. In the 2012 Olympics, Women's Boxing was officially recognized and approved for inclusion in the Games. History was made with world champion Katie Taylor fighting in arguably the best bout of the tournament (men or women). She fought a furious battle, so epic that it will long live in the memories of all who witnessed it, and emerged victorious. Make no mistake, boxing is a brutal sport, but if you would like to perfect your punching ability, have enhanced upper body power, as well as a great cardio workout, then women's boxing might be for you!

Crossfit - Crossfit is a strength and conditioning brand that combines weightlifting, gymnastics, and sprinting. It is the principal strength and conditioning program for many police academies, military special operations units, martial artists, specialized tactical units, and hundreds of other elite and professional athletes worldwide. Many gyms tailor their training routines to train combat and survival maneuvers. From the beginning, the aim of Crossfit has been to prepare trainees for any physical contingency—prepare them, not only for the known, but for the unknown. It develops a physical performance advantage to prepare the trainee for almost any physical obstacle. Most monsters are in terrible shape (drugs and alcohol do not do a body good). Crossfit workouts are typically short but intense, demanding an all-out physical effort. I recommend this as a very viable self defense option because the types of exercises that are done use muscles not routinely used in other training styles. Crossfit employs some very unorthodox exercises, such as swinging objects – axes and other sticks, in ways to strengthen muscle groups that will help you deliver some very effective strikes if needed. Your legs will become powerfully strong and your endurance level will be greater. If you need to kick someone and run, chances are he won't be able to keep up with you in the long haul. An extra benefit is that the physical transformation to your physique will be awesome.

"Only one who devotes himself to a cause with his whole strength and soul can be a true master. For this reason mastery demands all of a person."

-Albert Einstein

 Tae Kwon Do – Respect and courtesy, modesty, self-control, perseverance, indomitable spirit — Tae Kwon Do, the fighting form, is characterized by the extensive use of high standing and jump kicks as well as punches, and is practiced for sport, self-defense, and spiritual development. I'd like to add that it is much more than that. Tae Kwon Do is profound and philosophical. I walked into a school angry, full of self doubt, low self-esteem, and pain. The tough training I received helped me look past me and my pain and focus on meditation and discipline. Students learn the techniques of kicking, punching, and blocking, which are practiced in a combined series of movement sets or forms. The word "Tae" "Kwon" "Do" is composed of three parts as - "Tae" means "foot," "leg," or "to step on"; "Kwon" means "fist," or "fight"; and "Do" means the "way" or "discipline." Tae Kwon Do strives to develop the positive aspects of an individual's personality: respect, courtesy, goodness, trustworthiness, loyalty, humility, courage, patience, integrity, perseverance, self control, an indomitable spirit, and a sense of responsibility to help and respect all forms of life. However, it is the physical, mental, and spiritual effort that the individual puts forth that develops the positive attributes and image of both the individual and how he or she perceives others. Ronda (3rd Dan Black Belt) describes, "It is a deep and meaningful art of introspection and finding a positive way to interact with others – benefiting you and them."

⬧ Karate – Karate, also known as the "empty hand", is the unarmed martial-arts discipline of employing kicks, strikes, and defensive blocks with arms and legs. "Karate-do" literally means "the way of the empty hand". The art is rooted in deep philosophical and spirited traditions based on Zen Buddhist principles. Karate is meant to not only strengthen the body, but also the mind and spirit. The Japan Karate Association eloquently describes the beauty and intensity of the art form. Emphasis of training is on focusing as much of the body's power as possible at the point of impact. Striking surfaces include the hands, ball of the foot, heel, forearm, knee, and elbow. Timing, tactics, and spirit, however, are each considered at least as important as physical toughening. It is more than a martial art. It is a way of life that trains a practitioner to be peaceful; but if conflict is unavoidable, true karate dictates taking down an opponent with a single blow. Such an action requires strength, speed, focus, control. But these physical aspects are only part of the practice; they are just the vehicle, not the journey itself. In true karate, the body, mind, and spirit — the whole person — must be developed simultaneously. Through kihon, kumite and kata a practitioner learns to control her movements. She can perform the techniques without thinking about them, and remain focused without having to concentrate on any one thing. In essence, the body remembers how to move and the mind remembers how to be still. This harmonious unity of mind and body is intensely powerful. The result of true karate is natural, effortless action, and the confidence, humility, openness and peace only possible through perfect unity of mind and body. This is the core teaching of Zen, the basis of Bushido, and the central focus of the JKA's karate philosophy. The foundation of karate is the kihon (basic techniques), the kata (forms), and the kumite (sparring). Upon these three rest all technique, all speed, all strength and all progress in karate. They are, in essence, one. And they must be studied as one: without the kihon basic techniques, there can be neither kata nor kumite. Likewise, kata separated from kumite is simply rote movement unseasoned with the knowledge that comes from application. Finally, kumite without kata loses the characteristic agility and effortless smoothness inherent in karate. Kihon is kata is kumite. Appreciating that there is value in a style of fighting other than just kicking and punching is an added bonus to becoming fearless. There is so much history and beauty to learn in this craft.

There are so many wonderful and effective methods of self defense. Each one has its own unique points. Aside from the ones I chose to showcase here, there are other very effective styles. I encourage you to take the step to developing a strong mind and body. The benefits are endless. You will be in better shape, learn defensive skills, practice peaceful centered meditation, and become part of a team. Go for it, Girl!

Understand that most beasts have no training at all. Their secret weapon in an attack is fear and intimidation. They know if they get you by surprise, you will be easier to overcome.

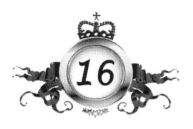

The Wicked Punch

Strikes

"Fear of the punch is worse than the reality of the punch"

- Cathy

If there is no easy escape from a bad situation, I want you to know and understand that the fear of a strike is much worse than the actual strike itself. Many of us see movies and TV shows that depict being hit as something so painful we will instantly be incapacitated. Although, if Mike Tyson were to strike you with a hay-maker, it would definitely be painful (or not, because you will be knocked out and won't feel a thing), most attacks I have studied aren't at the level of a trained fighter. Most attackers are counting on your fear to beat you. Don't get me wrong; it will hurt, maybe not at the moment because your adrenaline will be pumping, but you will feel it once the event is over, you are safe, and you have calmed down.

Understand that most beasts have no training at all. Their secret weapon in an attack is fear and intimidation. They know if they get you by surprise, you will be easier to overcome. In most attacks, women usually freeze with fear and cower in a standing fetal position covering their faces and head as if their spindly arms and hands could shield a blow. This is a mistake. You need to be bobbing and weaving. Move! Look alive. You are a strong woman and are not going to make yourself a punching bag.

Stand up with your knees slightly bent, your fist up, and be ready to deflect. Punch, scratch, gouge, palm strike, elbow, or do anything you can to get an opening so you can run!

Remember one thing, no matter if it works effectively or not: kicking the groin is the first thing your attacker will expect. Not to say if you have a clear opening you shouldn't take it. Keep in mind the body has many areas that could cause enough injury to make the attacker stop – even if momentarily to give you a window of escape. Once you have achieved your escape, run, scream, make yourself unstoppable, and get away.

Here are a few moves I want you to practice and know:

- Palm Strikes – Palm strikes seem like they are so girlie, but, trust me, a good palm strike can ring someone's bell when delivered with force. Press your fingers tightly together and slap the side of his head on his ear. Imagine yourself trying to hit the opposite ear by using enough force to penetrate through his skull, by imagining that you will instinctively strike with greater force. If you see the object you are striking as the final stop, you will recoil your hand too quickly and the hit will not be as effective. Try it for yourself. First, strike a pillow propped up on your bed. Then strike the bed through the pillow. You will inevitably strike the pillow harder the second time to have enough force to get through the pillow in order to hit the bed….. You should practice all your strikes this way.

↗ Heel palm strikes are very effective. Take your hand and position it like you are indicating someone to stop. The bottom of your hand is the heel. Use the heel of your hand to strike your attacker's nose. Thrust your hand upwards straight from your chest and strike the nose right at the nostrils. P.A.I.N.F.U.L.! Then run! The nose has many nerve endings at the base of the nostrils, and the nasal passage is connected to the eyes via the tear ducts. Therefore, if you cause trauma to the nose, the eyes will respond by welling up with water. Another great strike is to thrust your hand forward and hit him in the center of the chest over the heart. Every strike you deliver is done with absolute force.

↗ Perfect Punch – Punches are pretty tricky. An effective punch requires precision, accuracy, and force. I have seen a video of a relatively small girl level a guy with one wild punch but it was pure luck. I don't want to lure you into a false sense of security thinking that going toe to toe with your beast is a good, viable option, unless you have had training (extensive training). There are a few "buttons" on a face that, if hit properly, will knock out an opponent. The ability to master the strike necessary to hit them requires training and luck. One big issue with a closed fist punch is that your hands have a series of thin brittle bones that line the outside of your hand, connecting at your knuckles. If you punch someone incorrectly, you run a great risk of breaking the bones in your

"I fear not the man who has practiced 10,000 kicks once, but I fear the (Wo)man who has practiced one kick 10,000 times"

-Bruce Lee

hand. Now you are out of the fight. You are mentally and physically preoccupied with the pain. Your asset is your quick wit and brain and now it is overloaded with messages of pain from your hand. You need to stay sharp and constantly thinking in order to escape this event. Don't default to swinging a traditional punch unless you have trained extensively on how to effectively throw it. If you are not trained, then I suggest trying one of two punches I call perfect.

The throat punch – curl your fingers like you are about to knock on a door, tuck your thumb on the outside of the curled fingers (Never tuck your thumb in the fold of your fingers.), then shoot your arm straight out and strike the throat or the side of the neck. You need to hit like you are trying to reach a door behind him.

When he grabs his throat, gasping for air and looking at you in horror, run! You have stunned him and he might not go after you, but then again, he might, so run like the wind, screaming like a banshee.

Solar Plexus shot – The solar plexus is located right beneath the spot where your ribs meet, just above your belly button. Ball up your hand into a fist, again being careful about the placement of your thumb, and shoot it forward, hitting him right in the meaty spot. That area houses the diaphragm, which helps us breathe. Delivering a blow to this muscle causes great pain and a harsh reaction such as vomiting or loss of breath — and again, gives you that free second to run away. Ronda recommends the Hammer Fist as a great alternative to a punch, and I will have to agree. As the name suggests, you are using the fist as a hammer to strike. The part of the hand that will be used to strike will be the side of your pinkie. "You can swing down and at an angle into the soft tissues around the neck with quite a bit of force. Since you're using a hammer fist, the pain you may feel will be minimal; even if you miss and hit the collar bone or shoulder, they will likely still feel a good deal of pain, and if your adrenaline is helping to propel your strike, you may get lucky and break the collar bone. The great thing about a hammer fist is how many directions you can swing from: from high coming straight down with or without an angle, you can swing out to the side as well and it still has a powerful swing." Swing your hammer fist and strike the temple of the head or right around the eye sockets. This will deliver a serious blow that will ring his bell for a little while. While he tries to remember where he is at, run! Furiously swing your hammer fist at his jaw. Remember the "buttons" I mentioned; the jaw is a major knock-out point. A good wallop on his jaw could send him straight to the ground.

- Elbow Strikes – Elbow strikes happen to be my favorite striking method. Your elbow could be used as a baton. If you are face to face and in close proximity with your attacker, sweep your elbow in an upward motion, striking under the jaw. Ouch! That hit will jar even the toughest of men who aren't expecting that kind of force being delivered by what they thought was going to be an easy victim. A good upward elbow to the jaw could cause some serious damage to teeth and tongue, as well as a whiplash he won't forget in the morning. Straight backward elbow – If he comes up behind you and applies a bear hug to carry you into his car, bend your arm at a 90 degree angle, move your arm forward to try to break his grip then thrust it backwards into his ribs, stomach, or solar plexus. That should get his attention. If he grabs your arm from behind, swing it forward to try to break his grip, spinning the other way with an elbow to the head or face with your free arm. OK, now he is thinking he may have bitten off more than he could chew. A sideways elbow across his jaw or eye is exceptionally effective if your attacker is close to you. Lift your fist to your neck, raise your elbow, and swing at his jaw or eye. Notice that your strike zone is small, so he must be close for you to reach. Put your body into it. Use the force of your whole body when you hit someone with an elbow.

⬧ Kicks and knees- The use of kicks and knees could be a very powerful tool to a woman. The strongest muscles in our body are our quadriceps (thighs). With the help of strong leg muscles, hips, and the huge leg bones, we could deliver a pretty potent strike. The first and very obvious kick or knee strike on an aggressor would be the groin. You should note that although it is VERY effective, most, if not all, men will instantly guard their groin region first. It's like second nature. It is their kryptonite. A swift kick to the groin of even the biggest monster will cause him great agony. If there is an opening, by all means take it, but don't fixate on that kick alone. Kick the side of his knee or the front of his knee. The knee is a vulnerable spot that will cause his leg to buckle and keep him from being able to effectively chase you. All you need, is to strike the side of his knee with the top of your foot with brutal force. To hit the front of his knee, bring up your knee slightly and shoot your foot forward with your toes back, and strike with the ball of your foot. The ball is the meaty part on the under-side of your foot (just below your toes). Use the force you would need if you were breaking down a door. Knee strikes are very effective with practice. It takes a short distance gap and allows for you to employ a powerful defense. You must lean into the strike with your whole body. That's the trick. The three main whoppers of knee strikes are the Charlie horse knee, the gut shot, and the head shot. The Charlie Horse is a difficult one to execute flawlessly without practice. It is taking a shot at the monster's outer thigh with your knee. The nerve that runs along the outer part of the leg will cause his leg to spasm if applied properly. The gut shot is executed by grabbing his shoulders, pulling him forward and into you, then bursting towards him in an explosion of power using your whole body to deliver the hit with your knee. The head shot is applied if he is already leaning forward, because you caused him to bend forward with a previous strike. Grab his head or shirt collar and strike with your knee. I suggest you knee the under part of the jaw, the side temple or side of his face. Try to avoid kneeing the front of his face; although it seems like a good move, you could possibly injure your knee and soft muscle tissue above your knee with teeth and the bones of the nose. Deliver your strikes with short, powerful bursts using your body weight for maximum effect.

- Finger poke (no manicures will be ruined in practice) – A Monster cannot attack what he cannot see. Just as the name suggests, you are looking to poke your attacker. You poke him in the eyes with your finger. It doesn't have to be both eyes, as one will be just as effective. If you are like me, the thought of sticking your finger in someone's gooey eye will give you goose bumps. The first time I put contacts in my eyes, I almost fainted just looking at my finger closing in on my eyeball. You need to make him want to retreat and get away from you so you drive that finger into his gooey eyeball and make it count. Grab his head and use your thumbs to press in his eyes. Again, just typing that makes me nauseous, but it is necessary to get him to draw back his attack on you.

"Every time I get an eyelash or a micro-scopic piece of sand in my eye, I'm practically useless until it gets cleaned out. Now, if you hate getting those tiny things in your eyes - imagine how debilitating it can be to have someone's fingers jammed into the eye(s)."

Ronda Fleites
3rd Dan Black Belt

Take your finger and ram it up his nostril then hook it and scratch the inside of his nose while pulling your finger free. Trust me — this will be so painful, his eyes will water and he will loos-

en his grip on you. The nose is very sensitive and has many nerve endings. Any kind of strike to the nose will have even the most relentless beast think twice about whether this attack was a good idea or not.

In a panic, if all else fails and you can't think

straight, just go wild and scratch his face at the eyes. If he is so daring as to attack, you need to make him regret it as quickly as possible, to make him leave you alone and not give chase when you run away.

 Stomps of Pain – Feet have many small brittle bones working in unison to allow you to walk and run. If someone grabs you from behind, stomp your heel into the top of their foot, right at the hump, a few inches above their toes. Do it as many times as you can. Use the force necessary to reach through and touch the ground. Grind down like you are putting out a dirty cigarette with your heel. I can pretty much guarantee he isn't going to be chasing you anywhere, Fabulous. I'd be surprised if he could even walk after such a counterattack. Another very painful kind of stomp is, if he has grabbed you from behind, take the heel of your foot and scrape it down the front of his leg, below the knee. This area is called the shin. The shin is just the tibia bone covered in a thin layer of skin. Drag your heel down the shin and end it with a ferocious stomp that will make him see stars. That momentary blink offers you a head start to escape his attack.

"If you know the enemy and know yourself you need not fear the results of a hundred battles."

-Sun Tzu

- Hair Pulling – Pulling hair is so primitive, but highly effective in taking your monster off balance. Where the head goes, the body will follow. Grab a chunk of hair and pull it down with the force of the weight of your entire body. Yank it with a furious jerking motion. The only thing holding that miserable head in place is a skinny neck, so go crazy. This method only works if your beast has hair. Baldies could be a problem.

- The Bite – If your foolish beast decides to cover your mouth to prevent you from screaming, then bite his hand. Bite so hard you take his skin off. Don't stop until your upper and lower teeth touch. If he thought trying to shut you up by covering your mouth was a good idea, then show him how it might have been better if he had stayed in bed this morning. You are not one to be played with. You are fierce and will fight with everything you have to protect your awesome peaceful life.

- Pinkie Promise – This Pinkie will be broken, I promise! This is an awesome technique to break a hold your beast has on you. It is so easy to apply. If your monster has hold of you, while wrestling with him in your effort to get away, try and grab hold of his pinkie. Once you have the pinkie in hand – slam the finger to the outside of his hand. Try to make it touch his wrist. Test out the limits of pain on yourself, so you can best determine which way to bend it to get the quickest response. Practice carefully and slowly with a friend to test the breaking sweet spot.

This way, in your mind you already know how far you have to go to get it done. You definitely don't want to stop too early and just sting your attacker, allowing him a quick recovery and to resume attacking you. You have to remove all doubt from his mind that he should leave you alone. Note that hand strength is greater closer to the thumb, but it doesn't mean all is lost if you happen to grab hold of another finger in your struggle. Test out each one of your finger's threshold of pain. Chances are, when your adrenaline is high, you could break any one of them with the right force. Practice. You are making yourself your own heroine! Every Fabulous heroine has to have several signature moves. Remember to not get fixated trying a move you can't finish. This is a move of opportunity. If he doesn't give up his hand right away, move on to something else. Verse yourself in several moves. Keep your mind sharp and thinking while the attack is in motion. As the events unfold, decide how you are going to respond. Your real priority is looking to escape.

Realize that every opportunity to escape is crucial to your survival. If you get lucky with a perfectly executed strike that leaves your monster incapacitated for a moment, DO NOT decide to try to finish him off with more strikes. You are not a ninja, and unless you have lots of training to back you up, I suggest you take that opening to get yourself to safety. Practice these moves at home and with friends. Repeating the motions effectively over and over will commit them to muscle memory. Muscle memory is your instinctive physical response to a situation. Just as you have certain movements you do naturally because you have done them so many times in your life, the same can happen with defensive moves.

If you feel inspired, I would love to see you in a martial arts class. It made all the difference in my life, and I know you would learn so much about yourself, what you are actually capable of with the right training, and confidence. All I see is a win-win.

Keep your options open when confronted by a monster. See the potential in everything. The simplest-looking object can be effective to help you escape a monster. Open your mind.

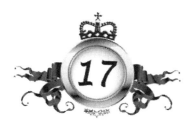

Fabulously Fierce!

Weapons

Bare handed strikes and kicks can be pretty effective as diversionary tactics to get away from an attack. You should have the ability to identify potential weapons at your disposal for the occasion when those tactics just aren't enough. When your monster is completely fixated on the fact that you are going to be his victim, you need to quickly react with extreme accuracy in order to survive. This chapter will cover many different types of weapons and also help you see the potential of everyday items as weapons. Your quick identification and reaction could be the difference between your beautiful life now, a damaged existence, or possibly death. Let's rock!

> *"Above all, be the heroine of your life, not the victim"*
> *- Nora Ephron*

Fiercely Effective:

- Guns – I used to fear guns. As with most things we don't know much about, I just thought they were dangerous and could unpredictably discharge. The first time I held a gun, my biggest fear was if it would go off accidentally, and I would hurt or kill someone. The first time I squeezed the trigger, the loud bang and power of the recoil flung my hands back, causing me to jump in fear and almost drop it. I kept my fear suppressed, and I shot again and again until the magazine was empty and pulling the trigger yielded no results. When I saw my target dotted with the holes in the general area where I was aiming, it felt good. I kept coming back to the range to practice and build my confidence. I also did simulation training. Sim training is done with a laser gun and computer generating scenarios where you have to make split-second decisions on whether to shoot or not. It tries to replicate the real world with sights and sounds to make your adrenaline start pumping. Guns come in a range of sizes to fit small hands and large ones. The calibers of guns range from .22 mini guns to .50 caliber hand cannons. You will definitely find a gun perfectly suited for you if you choose to explore gun ownership. The small guns are a perfect fit for the petite purse or a small concealable holster worn on your body.

There are a few simple rules for safety when handling a gun:

1. Treat all firearms as if they are loaded - When you treat all weapons as if they are loaded, then you will always exercise extra caution when handling them.

2. Point the muzzle away from anything you don't intend to shoot – Seriously, in a moment of recklessness or panic, you could have your finger

in the wrong place and discharge your weapon. It happens, so just be careful.

3. Keep your fingers off the trigger – and I will add the trigger well — entirely. Triggers on most of these guns are highly reactive. If you touch them with some force, they will fire.

4. Be sure of your target, what is before it, and what is beyond it – Bullets sometimes miss their targets, so you need to be keenly aware of what is past your target. You don't want to hurt any-one or damage property by being irresponsible.

5. Practice – If you own a gun, you should practice regularly until you become proficient. There is no use owning a gun if you can't shoot it prop-erly. The main cause of injury at home is when the owner has minimal training or leaves a gun within reach of a child or person not properly trained in hand gun safety.

These rules are really straightforward. I added rule number 5 because, if you are going to be fierce, you have to actually know what you are doing. You wouldn't want to have to use your gun and miss your monster. Practice a few times. Become efficient and comfortable with the proper handling of a gun, and you will be glad you did if ever attacked. (For a more detailed discussion on women and guns, check out Kathy Jackson's book "*The Cornered Cat: A Woman's Guide to Concealed Carry*".)

⚐ Knives – Knives are pretty awesome. One of the oldest tools used by man, it has been used as both a tool and a weapon as far back as the stone ages. The earliest knives were made of stone, wood, ivory, and steel. Today, knives are made of different types of steel – stainless, carbon, and surgical — all extremely sharp and very durable. Knives come in all shapes and sizes. I am going to cover three types of knives for self defense — spring-loaded blades, push daggers, and finger hole knives. Note that certain knives are illegal in some states, so if you choose to explore ownership of one, you need to do your research.

Spring-assisted blade knife – This is a Fabulously fierce little weapon. The knife is safely tucked into its handle grip and accessed with the push of a button. The blade springs out into a locked position. I favor this knife because I have a daughter, and I fear if she reaches in my purse and pulls out a regular knife, she risks hurting herself. The activation button is very hard and requires some force to get it to open. Little hands will probably not be able to accidentally get it to the spring. Spring-loaded knives are classified as switchblades and are illegal in many states and countries.

Push Dagger – These little brutal blades are usually between two and four inches long with a T-shaped handle. The push dagger handle is held between your index and middle finger with the blade protruding outward. It swings in a forward manner, much like a punch. It is extremely effective in a close attack situation. There are several shapes and sizes available. I like the heart shaped one. Most come with a protective plastic or leather sleeve so you don't poke yourself when you put your hands into your purse.

Finger Hole knife – These are a short blade variety of knife. The blades come in different shapes and sizes. What is so appealing about these knives is that there are finger holes in the handle to secure your grip of the knife. I'm going to be honest; blood is slippery and if you are attacked and cut your monster, the knife could slip from your hand. It is important that you research not just the blade but the grip on the handle too. You don't want to risk being disarmed or your slippery knife sliding out of your hand in an attack. Try to never get a smooth grip handle. The reason behind that is so that if you need to quickly access the weapon and reach into your purse, the rougher texture will help you identify it by touch instead of having to look, keeping your eyes on your beast at all times to see what he is doing. Do your homework on what is legal in the state or country you live in to make sure you stay compliant with the law.

- Batons – Kubotans – Initially designed for female LAPD officers as a tool to restrain suspects without permanent injury, the kubotan is often touted as extremely effective in breaking the will of unruly suspects with painful locks and pressure point strikes. It is because of this that the kubotan has been dubbed the "Instrument of Attitude Adjustment." They are an extremely effective method of leveling the playing field when dealing with a larger and stronger attacker. Originally made of hard, high-impact plastic, the kubotan keychain is about 5.5 inches long and 0.56 inches in diameter. The kubotan is generally held in an ice pick (hammer fist) or forward stabbing grip. The most basic applications involve striking or poking vulnerable areas of the body with the kubotan. Generally speaking, swinging strikes work better against bony surfaces while fleshy areas are more susceptible to pokes and jabs with the ends of the kubotan. Basically, whatever it takes to ward off an attacker. A few common uses for the kubotan include hardening the fist for punching and gaining leverage on an attacker's wrist, fingers, and joints. Also, because the kubotan is small enough to attack anywhere the finger can, it can also be used for pressure point and pain compliance. Due to the size and shape of the kubotan, many of the self-defense techniques learned can be replaced by everyday items such as flashlights, pens, and markers, making the kubotan a very versatile weapon to own. The tip of the kubotan may either be pointed or flat. Thus, the effectiveness of this simple self defense instrument lies in the knowledge and skill of the person who will use it. If done effectively, it has the ability to temporarily paralyze or cause extreme pain to the attacker, allowing you more time to escape. The best places to attack when using the kubotan are the stomach, the groin, the solar plexus, the arm, the hip bone, the shin, the collarbone, the kneecap, the ankle, and the throat. An accurate attack on one of these body parts will certainly keep your assailant immobile for quite some time, but a more increased power strike may even lead to broken bones for your beast. If you are not sure about pressure points, the best moves you can make with a kubotan are the use of swinging strikes. It does not require any memorization of specific strikes and targets, except for the need to remember to poke soft tissues, strike bones and pressure points. Honestly, you can never go wrong with any strike using the kubotan. You simply need to hit as hard as you can because the material used in creating the kubotan is sufficient to aid your every blow. Jab your kubotan into someone's ribs, solar plexus, or back to reinforce your position that No means No! Keep your kubotan close at all times. Unlike a gun, it is safe to keep anywhere without worry that a child could get hurt holding it. It is rather long, although it is usually between 5.5 – 7 inches, so you have to figure out where on your person you want to keep it for quick access. Remember that a weapon buried at the bottom of your purse or under your seat or glove compartment in your car is of no use to you. If you decide this is the best weapon for you, then you should figure out where to keep it readily available. It comes with a key ring at the end so it could be used as a flailing weapon to swing your keys at your monster's face. I would advise to use it for its intended nonlethal stabbing action. Oh, the pain this little unassuming stick will cause a foolish beast thinking you are an easy target.

- Pepper Spray – Pepper sprays are extremely effective as a nonlethal way to incapacitate your assailant, so you can escape. Measured in terms of capsaicoids, which is the degree of heat given off by a particular pepper, pepper spray is designed to cause your monster's eyes to slam shut and stay that way for a while. The secret is that it is a burning irritant and it sucks the tears right out of your eyes, making it virtually impossible for you to be able to naturally flush out the chemicals. This should render your beast almost useless for a few minutes. Even if he does get a hold of you, chances are he will not be very effective because the pain in his eyes will not be ignored. Pepper spray comes in several sizes and delivery systems. You could choose an aerosol cone or a gel stream delivery — they are both very effective. The aerosol cone is best deployed in an outdoor, well-ventilated area. You want to aim the spray right at the monster's face, focusing on his eyes for the best result. The spray has a natural orange color from the pepper, so it allows you to see exactly where you are hitting your target. The downside would be if you are inside a confined area, you could have what is referred to as a blow back. Blow back is when you deploy the spray and you get some of its effect. Not the situation you want to be in, so let me introduce you to the gel stream delivery method. The can sprays a stream of gel that reaches 10 feet. You want to aim right at the eyes and sweep side to side or ear to ear. The orange tint of the gel will let you know if you are on target or not. But if the orange gel stain on his face doesn't give you clear indication you've hit your mark, the flailing and eye-rubbing while yelling should make you feel confident you have effectively done your job. Run away and get help. Don't use this chance to go all crazy and start hitting him. You run the risk of exposing yourself to the effect of the pepper spray and will be right there beside him rubbing your eyes and screaming. The newest product in pepper spray technology is a blue dye that will stain the face for several days so, if your monster gets away, all police have to do is find the idiot with the blue-tinted face. That'll teach him to mess with a fiercely Fabulous girl!

- Stun Guns – Considered an Electroshock weapon, the simplest purpose of the stun gun is to disrupt the body's electrical system. The weapon delivers an electrical current to the body designed to incapacitate by causing muscles to seize up temporarily. The hand-held unit requires you to be in close contact with the attacker and place the unit against his body, keeping contact while activating the electrical pulse for several seconds.

Taser – Similar to the stun gun, but allows you to deploy spike prongs at a safe distance to activate the device and incapacitate your monster. The unit comes equipped with laser sights to very accurately aim at your approaching target. The prongs deliver an electrical current that disrupts voluntary muscle movement, momentarily incapacitating the monster. These electrodes create an unavoidable incapacitation that cannot be overcome. He WILL drop and stay that way for at least five seconds. Five seconds is all you need to make a run for it. Once you deploy the prongs and activate the taser, drop it and run. The company has a replacement policy. They will replace your unit with the proper paperwork – police report and purchase receipt. The downside of the taser is that if one of the prongs does not hit, then the circuit isn't complete, so the electrical jolt won't activate. In that case, you are required to press the taser against his body to shock him. Now you are in close contact, and once you let go, he has a pretty quick recovery.

NOTE: While the term "Taser" has been used generically in the above paragraph in reference to varying brands of Electronic Control Devices, it is important to note that "Taser" is a trademark of TASER International, Inc.

✓ Mini Air Horns – This is ear-piercing attention in a can. You have probably heard the high-pitched shriek of this horn at a sporting event and it inevitably caused your head to turn in the direction of the sound. It is almost impossible to ignore. Some people freeze up in high stress events. Their voice may fail them as well as the rest of their body. In an intensely stressful situation, the brain might identify the event but fail to send the proper signals to the body to respond appropriately in some people. The mini air horn can act as your voice and give you time to recover your reaction response, retrieve another weapon, or run to escape. These air horns come in a compact size. The alarm can be heard up to a quarter mile away. It is extremely loud. To activate it, you could press the button and hold it down for a long sustained blast or pump your finger several times to get several short bursts of ear-piercing shrieks. If I felt as if I were in danger of being attacked, I would take my air horn and blast it at my attacker. Actually, if he was upon me, I would take my horn, place it right against his head and discharge the screech right into his ear. He will walk away from this experience wishing he had stayed in bed that morning! My objective is to get away, but if my defense makes him re-evaluate his career choice in life, I'd be happy. It is a very nonlethal form of defense and possibly ineffective (if your monster is deaf) because it only deals in noise, which in essence only affects the ears. Don't get me wrong, a loud piercing sound will momentarily stun someone, but an attacker can still see you and chase you, even if his ears hurt. Understand, it is one of many choices for nonlethal defense.

- Keychain defense items – Kitty Keychain defense, breakaway key chain - there are several keychain defense items on the market. One extremely effective one is the kubotan I addressed earlier. One that can be extremely effective, also, and discreet, is the Kitty keychain. The Kitty keychain is in the shape of a cat face with holes for eyes large enough for you to insert your fingers and grip. The ears stick out and are effective for raking the outside of the hand of a beast who dares to lay a hand on you. You could do a number of things with the Kitty. You could rake the small bones on the outside of his hand if he grabs you, poke him with the ears in the ribs, rake the ribs, drive it into his neck, his eyes, nose, or mouth. Drive those little ears into his solar plexus and he will scream like a girl. A break-away key chain is a very valuable accessory to use. It separates your house key and car key rings with a detachable link. A break-away keychain is a must for the times when you take your car in for service and have to hand over your keys — unless you personally know the mechanic. You don't want them to have the keys to your home along with your car. In your car, the registration with your address is readily available. Actually, you probably gave them your address when you filled out the service request. Lots of mechanics shops make duplicate keys for a customer. A break away will let you detach your home keys and hand over the car keys and nothing more. A mini flashlight is a great weapon combo to have. It is functional in a bunch of ways. Aside from the obvious light uses, it could also be a modified kubotan. Grip your mini flashlight in your hand with the end protruding from your pinkie side and swing it like an ice pick! Poke, stab, and jab it into your monster's ribs, stomach, head, neck, eyes, arms, or back of the hands, to have him release his grip on you. An attacker will not take it easy on you, so return the favor to save your life.

- Everyday Items – Now that you are learning how to keep yourself safe in various situations, let's look at the common items around you. Start to look around your home to identify everyday items you could quickly grab in case of emergency to use as a weapon. What do you currently have by your front door that could be used to fight back a home invader attempting to enter your home? There are several pretty wall décor items available you could use to grab and stab, strike, or hit him with. You could set up a decorative shelf with a can of pepper spray, knife, or gun hidden on it for quick access. Keeping in mind the safety of those who live in your home and visitors with small children, and make sure it is at an appropriate height. What do you have at your bedside for protection? Perhaps a small heavy solid statue on your night stand will make a sweet weapon. Everyday household chemical sprays can deliver a nasty sting to the eyes of a monster if you are cornered and have no other choice. In your garden, a rock can be used to strike, dirt can temporarily blind someone, and a heavy branch could deliver a nasty blow! Look around now and familiarize yourself, so in an emergency, when your mind is racing, you don't have to think about it. You will just know.

Keep your options open when confronted by a monster. See the potential in everything. We sometimes get accustomed to thinking certain things need to look certain ways in order to be effective, and it's just not true. The simplest-looking object can be effective to help you escape a monster. Open your mind.

NOTE: Weapons laws vary from state to state. Before incorporating a weapon into your self defense system, I highly recommend you do some in-depth research to ensure you are following all federal, state and local weapons laws."

We are not meant to battle toe-to-toe with a man. We are made of a different fiber. While men specialize in brute force and muscle, we specialize in wit and cunning. It is our gift.

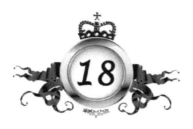

The Foolish Heroine

"Our wisdom comes from our experiences, and our experiences come from foolishness."

– *Sacha Guitry*

Training and the newfound sense of power can be intoxicating. Keep your wits about you, lady, and don't be a foolish heroine. I remember during a night out with girlfriends several years ago, we were walking along the street to our car after a fun night of dancing. I noticed a commotion behind us on the street as a Lexus screeched to a stop and two bald beefy body-builder types jumped out of the car and ran towards a scooter. On this scooter was an older man and a kid (somewhere around 12 years old). They began screaming at the old man and punched him, knocking him to the floor. I yelled "Hey!" as I started back towards them. The boy swung a wild punch but missed, and they punched him, also knocking him to the floor.

At this point I found myself running towards them screaming "Stop." They sprinted back to their car as I approached the boy to see if he was all right. He stumbled up to his feet with his one eye shut trying to get over to the old man as he lay on the ground. I was enraged and my inner heroine needed to get these guys. I whipped around and yelled, "Hey!" at them. When one of them looked back at me, I got in a fighting stance with my knees slightly bent, fists cocked up, and head slightly forward and said, "You punched this old man, you punched this kid, now come try your luck with a woman!" One of the guys said, "f*ck you b*tch!" After a dramatic look left, then right, I then replied, "I don't see who you're calling a b*tch." He stood there staring at me for a second. The other guy yelled "Come on, let's GO!" One more insult from the beef jerkies and they sped off.

I turned to check on the boy again when I noticed the crowd gathered around. I proceeded to call them cowards for not helping the old man and kid. I slowly strutted past the crowd glaring at them as I walked by. My girlfriends were pissed and rightfully so. What was I doing? At the moment I didn't think about the fact that if those two guys came back to fight I could have gotten hurt. Or that I just chastised a group of strangers – half of whom were drunk and possibly could have started a fight. At that moment I felt invincible. I was a warrior, a heroine. I was foolish.

"(S)He who knows when (s)he can fight and when (s)he cannot, will be victorious"

-Sun Tzu

Training and conditioning and the new self-confidence it brings will make you feel like you could suddenly right the wrongs of the world. Be smart. If something happens in your presence, call for help or get involved IF you absolutely must. My scenario was flawed because the threat to the old man and boy was over. The perpetrators were retreating. My new sense of strength and heroism clouded my judgment. Always remember this, girlie — with knowledge comes power and with power you can sometimes lose your focus and reason. Let the Fabulously fearless new you be centered and sensible.

Wit

"A witty woman is a treasure; a witty beauty is a power"

– George Meredith

Suffice to say, we are not built the same as men. We are not meant to battle toe-to-toe with a man. We are made of a different fiber. While men specialize in brute force and muscle, we specialize in wit and cunning. It is our gift. Use it to your advantage.

You, Fabulous, are special and perceptive. You see the world in various shades of possibilities and have the instinct to help you maneuver even the trickiest situations with sly craftiness. Your wonderful intuition will be your guide. Your astute awareness will help you see the first signs of danger, and your quick wit will help you figure out a way to quickly get away from it. Let your newfound knowledge help you realize that you have the greatest of gifts with your ability to quickly think on your feet. Be five steps ahead of the monstrous brute who wants to harm you. If he gets a hold of you, then use your keen skills to outwit him. Convince him with your charm that he needs to leave you alone. Although, if it doesn't work, I have provided you with a list of things you could do to physically get away from him. You are extremely capable of making a difference for yourself. Let your confidence shine.

"Go confidently in the direction of your dreams. Live the life you've imagined"

- Thoreau

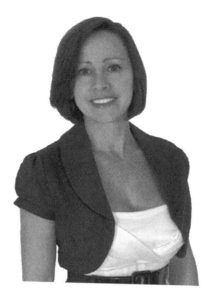

Cathy Steinberg is a black belt in Tae Kwon Do, an avid shooter, and former correctional officer at a maximum security male prison, a criminally insane mental hospital, and a death row women's prison - where she supervised infamous murderers like Judy "the Black Widow" Buenoano and Aileen Wournos - The first female serial killer.

Cathy is a personal safety expert and speaker who conducts safety workshops at all types of organizations and volunteers at local abuse shelters and nonprofit women's groups to teach personal safety, inspire and motivate women to take active roles in their self defense. She has dedicated her life to helping women lead safer lives.

Impact Statement

1 in 4 — two numbers that alone mean nothing, but the startling truth is that those numbers statistically determine that a woman's Fabulous existence will be decimated by a monster. He is out there lurking, waiting, and planning ways to hurt her. I know this monster intimately. He and I have met, and I know his mind, his thoughts, and his behaviors. He doesn't like me, because he knows I can help save you!

References

Tae Kwon Do

- Encyclopedia Britannica. Tae Kwon Do.
- Benko, Grand Master James S., Ph.D. The Philosophy of Tae Kwon Do.
- Fleites, Ronda. 3rd Dan Black Belt.
- World Tae Kwon Do Federation.
- Encyclopedia Britannica.

Krav Maga

- Krav Maga Federation
- Israeli Krav International

Jiu-Jitsu

- Encyclopedia Britannica
- Rousseau, Robert. A History and Style Guide to Jujitsu.
- Jiu-jitsu.net. The Advantages of Jiu-Jitsu

MMA

- Encyclopedia Britannica

Crossfit

- Glassman, Greg. The Crossfit Training Guide
- Crossfit.com. What is Crossfit?

Karate

- Encyclopedia Britannica
- Japan Karate Association. Forging a Karate Mind
- JKA. The Inseparable Trinity Lead to Kime

Kubotan

- Gorino, Master. Kubaton: Unassuming and Awesome Weapon by Master Gorino – Gorino Tae Kwon Do
- Breen, Andrew - The Kubaton

Other References

- Avant, Tamara. Examining Mob Mentality. South University, Savannah, GA. 2011
- Groth, Nicholas. Men Who Rape: The Psychology of the Offender. Basic Books. 1979
- Mann, Janice Lee; Ward, Diane; Westat. The Handbook for College Safety and Security Reporting, prepared for the Department of Education and The Office of Postsecondary Education
- Campus Safety and Security Data Analysis Cutting Tool. The Department of Postsecondary Education Reporting periods between 2008-10
- Jackson, Kathy - The Cornered Cat: A Woman's Guide to Concealed Carry
- Baum, Katrina PH.D.; Catalano, Shannan PH.D.; and, Michael – Bureau of Justice Statistics, Rose, Kristina – National Institute of Justice. Stalking Victimization in the United States
- Black, Michele C.; Basile, Kathleen C.; Breiding, Matthew J.; Smith, Sharon G.; Walters, Mikel L.; Merrick, Melissa T.; Chen, Jieru; Stevens, Mark R. CDCP – The National Intimate Partner and Sexual Violence Survey 2010

Acknowledgements

Loving thank you to my Padrino for sticking by me and Gale, Debbie, Matt, Joe, Ronda, Gabby, Joseph, Robert and kids – Love you!

Te quiero Tio Felo, Bidy, Jim and Cristina.

A special thanks to my oldest and dearest friends who have loved me and stood by me even when I used to throw chairs and fight with them. Adita, Michy, Adry, Maylin, Liz, Arlene, Carmel, Annette, Adri, Patty, Alex, Carlos, Ralph and crew. Love you guys. Your friendship got me through the toughest time in my life.

A heartfelt thank you to Liz Jurjo – my Angel who changed my life by introducing me to martial arts. You have no idea how you made a difference in my life. I am forever in your debt.

Thank you bunches to the most amazing girlfriends a person could ever wish for – DeeDee, Jenni, Jill, Jodi, Lori, Sara who welcomed me into their tribe. Extra special thanks to Jodi for reviewing it and giving me extra push to do it, Sara for using her expert talent to polish it up, and Jenni for promoting it.

Thank you to the fabulously awesome girlfriends who couldn't be more fun and supportive if they tried – Ali, Carol, Cynthia, Farah, Jenny, Ildi, Karen, Naydu, Nicole, and Mary

Thank you to Skip Coryell and Family at White Feather Press for giving me a chance. Buckle up it's gonna be a long ride!

18265342R00107

Made in the USA
Charleston, SC
25 March 2013